NEW DIRECTIONS FOR MENTAL HEALTH SERVICES

H. Richard Lamb, *University of Southern California*
EDITOR-IN-CHIEF

New Developments in Psychiatric Rehabilitation

Arthur T. Meyerson
Hahnemann University

Phyllis Solomon
Hahnemann University

EDITORS

Number 45, Spring 1990

JOSSEY-BASS INC., PUBLISHERS
San Francisco • Oxford

New Developments in Psychiatric Rehabilitation.
Arthur T. Meyerson, Phyllis Solomon (eds.).
New Directions for Mental Health Services, no. 45.

NEW DIRECTIONS FOR MENTAL HEALTH SERVICES
H. Richard Lamb, Editor-in-Chief

NEW DIRECTIONS FOR MENTAL HEALTH SERVICES is part of The Jossey-Bass Social and Behavioral Sciences Series and is published quarterly by Jossey-Bass Inc., Publishers (publication number USPS 493-910). Second-class postage paid at San Francisco, California, and at additional mailing offices. Postmaster: Send address changes to Jossey-Bass Inc., Publishers, 350 Sansome Street, San Francisco, California 94104.

EDITORIAL CORRESPONDENCE should be sent to the Editor-in-Chief, H. Richard Lamb, Department of Psychiatry and the Behavioral Sciences, U.S.C. School of Medicine, 1934 Hospital Place, Los Angeles, California 90033.

Library of Congress Catalog Card Number LC 87-646993

International Standard Serial Number ISSN 0193-9416

International Standard Book Number ISBN 1-55542-832-0

Cover Photograph by Wehrner Krutein/PHOTOVAULT.

Manufactured in the United States of America. Printed on acid-free paper.

Contents

Editors' Notes

The field of psychiatric rehabilitation has received increasing acceptance as a viable treatment approach for those who have severe mental disabilities. Psychiatric rehabilitation professionals, guided by an optimistic attitude, believe that professional interventions encompassing social, coping, and instrumental skill training and modification of physical and social environments of those with psychiatric disabilities can produce significant improvements in functioning and quality of life (Liberman and others, 1987; Anthony and Liberman, 1986), Thus, psychiatric rehabilitation is directed at changing the behaviors of psychiatrically disabled persons as well as the systems in which they live, learn, and work (Anthony and Liberman, 1986). The current philosophy and ideology of the field is one of building on an individual's strengths and believing that patients and clients can "learn, grow, and change" (Modrcin, Rapp, and Poertner, 1988; Harding and others, 1987).

Psychiatric rehabilitation professionals can no more afford to maintain a closed mind than to maintain the locked wards of institutions. Rather, they must open both their minds and the institutional doors to creative programming that is responsive to client needs. The field can no longer be confined to hospitals and agencies but needs to use the community and other systems as resources to obtain what clients need and want. In this context, research is a tool for change that ensures psychiatric professionals that their programs and systems are best serving clients.

The purpose of this volume is twofold: to describe several program models and approaches to psychiatric rehabilitation and to describe experimental efforts directed at modifying system and program environments to meet the needs of severely mentally disabled persons. The volume presents exciting conceptions of psychiatric rehabilitation and creative research and funding strategies that impact systems and programs.

Chapter One presents a detailed discussion of comprehensive biological-behavioral-psychosocial treatment approaches, including the UCLA prescriptive approach. Chapters Two and Three deal with research efforts directed at modifying the Social Security System for individuals who are severely mentally disabled. Chapters Four and Five address recently expanded opportunities in employment programming, including supportive employment and transitional employment. A creative funding strategy for developing housing alternatives for persons who have severe mental disabilities is presented in Chapter Six. This is followed by a discussion of The Robert Wood Johnson Foundation's program of funding innovative services for meeting the needs of persons with severe mental illness (Chapter Seven). Finally, Chapter Eight offers an approach to incorporating research into a psychosocial rehabilitation program whose components can be adapted in whole or in part.

The editors hope that this volume will stimulate a wider application of these efforts as well as the creation of other innovative models and strategies for policy and program change. Further, we implore the reader to incorporate research into these efforts. Without sound evidence for psychiatric rehabilitation, we may find that it neither flourishes nor survives the political and economic constraints the field is encountering. Similarly, without sound evidence for policy changes and developments, we will have little impact. We start by applauding our contributors, who included research in their efforts, and we entreat those who did not to do so.

References

Anthony, W. A., and Liberman, R. P. "The Practice of Psychiatric Rehabilitation: Historical, Conceptual and Research Base." *Schizophrenia Bulletin,* 1986, *12* (4), 542-559.

Harding, C., Brooks, G., Ashikaga, T., Strauss, J. S., and Breier, A. "The Vermont Longitudinal Study of Persons with Severe Mental Illness. I: Methodology, Study Sample, and Overall Status 32 Years Later." *American Journal of Psychiatry,* 1987, *144* (6), 718-726.

Liberman, R. P., Jacobs, H. E., Blackwell, G., Simpson, A., and Massel, H. K. "Overcoming Psychiatric Disability Through Skills Training." In A. T. Meyerson and T. Fine (eds.), *Psychiatric Disability: Clinical, Legal, and Administrative Dimensions.* Washington, D.C.: American Psychiatric Press, 1987.

Modrcin, M., Rapp, C., and Poertner, J. "The Evaluation of Case Management Services with the Chronically Mentally Ill." *Evaluation and Program Planning,* 1988, *11,* 307-314.

Arthur T. Meyerson is chair and professor in the Department of Mental Health Sciences, Hahnemann University.

Phyllis Solomon is professor and director of the Section of Mental Health Services and Systems Research, Department of Mental Health Sciences, Hahnemann University.

Comprehensive psychiatric rehabilitation for severely disabled patients must incorporate both biological and behavioral-psychosocial treatment approaches, applied over time in a range of community and institutional treatment settings.

Prescriptive Rehabilitation for Severely Disabled Psychiatric Patients

Mark L. Schade, Patrick W. Corrigan, Robert P. Liberman

Schizophrenia is a complex disease with numerous models describing etiology, phenomenology, and treatment. Two research agendas dominate. Biological approaches focus on neurochemistry and anatomy, whereas psychological approaches emphasize environmental stressors, diminished social and coping skills repertoires, and limited support systems. Psychiatric rehabilitation has been defined as the facilitation of the "physical, emotional, and intellectual skills needed to live, learn, and work in the community" (Anthony and Liberman, 1986, p. 542). However, the refractoriness of a large number of patients requires the implementation of rehabilitative methods based on the breadth of knowledge regarding schizophrenic functioning and deficits. Such an integrative approach can be achieved only through an interaction of both biological and environmental agendas.

The stress-diathesis model integrates physiological and behavioral aspects of schizophrenia (Nuechterlein and Dawson, 1984a; Zubin and Spring, 1977). As a result of genetic anomalies (Gottesman, McGuffin, and Farmer, 1987), persons with schizophrenia develop a range of psy-

The authors wish to thank Charles Wallace, Thad Eckman, Timothy Kuehnel, and Gayla Blackwell of the Camarillo/UCLA Clinical Research Center for Schizophrenia and Psychiatric Rehabilitation and Helene Lome, Ruth Davies-Farmer, James Stavish, and Richard Haar of First Step.

chophysiological and cognitive deficits that typically emerge in subclinical form during adolescence or young adulthood. Persons with schizophrenia demonstrate anomalous functioning on smooth-pursuit eye movement tasks, conduction of electric current through the skin, EEG alpha activity, heart rate, and blood pressure (Dawson and Nuechterlein, 1984). Skin conductance, heart rate, and blood pressure findings suggest that persons with schizophrenia suffer from aberrant arousal patterns, which may contribute to their hypersensitivity to stress.

Numerous information-processing deficits have been identified as well. Limits in functioning have been identified in sustained attention (Nuechterlein, 1977), iconic memory (Sacuzzo, 1986), long-term recall (Koh, 1978), and response selection (Broen, 1968). Nuechterlein and Dawson (1984b) have explained these dysfunctions in terms of Kahneman's (1973) finite-capacity view of information processing, suggesting that persons with schizophrenia have insufficient capacity for allocation to appropriate cognitive stages to sustain normal information processing. Aberrant arousal patterns may exacerbate deficits in information processing, since available capacity sharply declines in hyperaroused states (Gjerde, 1983).

The combination of diminished cognitive capacity and tonic aroused states is likely to accelerate vulnerability to environmental stress such that an increase in psychotic symptoms results when the low stress threshold is exceeded. Relapse is closely associated with a stressful life experience in the weeks before symptom exacerbation (Birley and Brown, 1970; Brown and Birley, 1968; Brown, Harris, and Peto, 1973). Furthermore, these stressful experiences are not clearly independent of the influence of the disease (Lukoff, Snyder, Ventura and Nuechterlein, 1984). Low tolerance for stress and periods of acute symptomatology combine to increase the frequency and severity of stressful life events. For example, Brown and Birley (1968) found that 40 percent of their patient sample were involved in legal proceedings, made long-distance moves, or changed jobs in the period prior to relapse.

Biological vulnerabilities and environmental response to stressors interact to affect the patient's repertoire and support network. Poor cognitive abilities are likely to impede sufficient acquisition of social and coping skills during prodromal years. As a result, the patient may be more exposed to social stressors and unable to accomplish instrumental goals. The combination of diminished coping skills and physiological sensitivity to arousal promotes avoidance of mildly stressful social situations. Similarly, the volatile course of the disease typically brings about estrangement from family, friends, neighbors, and co-workers, thus depriving the individual of an important "stress buffer."

The stress-diathesis model suggests that rehabilitation research and treatment requires interaction of biological and psychological views of the illness. In support of this model, drug and psychosocial treatment have been found to have synergistic effects (Falloon and Liberman, 1983; Liberman, Corrigan, and Schade, 1989). In one study, drug therapy reduced hospitalization rates to 41 percent; social skills training added to neuroleptic administrations reduced rates to 20 percent. When social skills training, behavior family management, and drug therapy were combined, *none* of the patients were found to be hospitalized at follow-up (Anderson, Reiss, and Hogarty, 1986).

Implications for Rehabilitation

A comprehensive, biological-psychosocial treatment approach can be described by means of a decision tree for the clinical management of schizophrenic patients (Liberman, Falloon, and Wallace, 1984). In this empirically informed approach, illustrated in Figure 1, patient characteristics and treatment needs provide a rationale for applying a broad range of psychosocial and neuroleptic drug interventions. Initial treatment efforts emphasize stress reduction, supportive use of the environment, and pharmacotherapy directed toward alleviating florid psychotic symptoms, particularly those that interfere with the patient's capacity to process information, voluntarily collaborate in treatment planning, and actively engage in psychosocial rehabilitation.

A tiny subgroup of patients may benefit from a drug-free trial of treatment. However, candidates for drug-free treatment of schizophrenia should pass a highly restrictive set of screening criteria, including having a first acute onset of symptoms with prominent affective components and clear precipitating events; having good premorbid social and occupational adjustment; living with relatives who are low in expressed criticism and hostility; being free of paranoid ideation; having realistic, integrative, and insightful attitudes regarding schizophrenia; and reporting dysphoric subjective response to a test dose of a neuroleptic, which may predict poor compliance with medication (Liberman, Falloon, and Wallace, 1984). For most patients, initial treatment will include neuroleptic drug therapy combined with goal-oriented, practical psychosocial treatment aimed at crisis intervention. Whether or not the initial, ordinarily brief (two-week to two-month) period of acute treatment takes place in a hospital, day treatment center, home-based setting, or other community setting will depend on the availability of nonhospital settings and resources and the supportive capacity of the family (Liberman, Falloon, and Wallace, 1984).

When the patient is relatively free of acute positive symptoms and cognitive dysfunction, a flexible psychosocial rehabilitation program can be instituted, in conjunction with continued administration of judicious doses of maintenance antipsychotic medications. Rehabilitation programs

Figure 1. Decision Tree for Clinical Management of Schizophrenia: Drug and Psychosocial Treatment Strategies

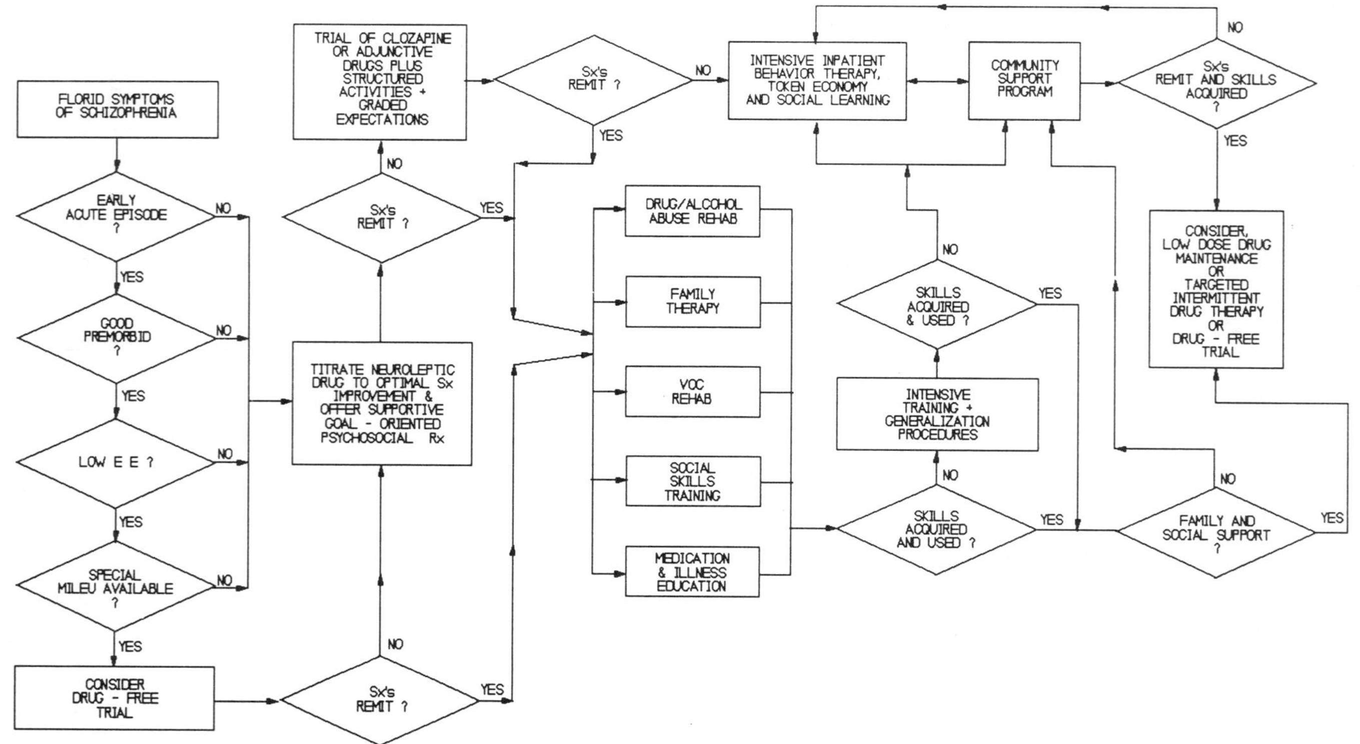

are graded, long-term, and aimed at remedying those behavioral deficits that remain after remission of florid symptoms. Rehabilitation also promotes drug compliance, with the goal of enabling patients to live in the community for longer periods of time without symptom exacerbation or rehospitalization.

For the approximately 60 to 70 percent of patients who remain in relative remission for one year after their last relapse and hospitalization, an important clinical decision becomes how long to continue medication. Recent studies found that remissions lasted longer among patients maintained on long-acting depot neuroleptics than among those maintained on oral medications, suggesting that long-term compliance with medication is an important element in rehabilitation (Hogarty and others, 1988). Combining behavioral training of patients in appropriate long-term use of antipsychotic medication—including knowing the benefits, side effects, techniques of self-administration, and how to negotiate medication issues with health care providers—can foster better outcomes from maintenance therapy (Eckman, Liberman, Phipps, and Blair, 1989). It is becoming increasingly apparent that neuroleptic drugs delay but rarely prevent relapse; hence, clinicians might consider lowering dose levels during maintenance periods in an effort to reduce the hazards of tardive dyskinesia and other long-term side effects (Liberman, Falloon, and Wallace, 1984). Moreover, one strategy that can compensate for the symptom breakthroughs experienced by patients on low-dose neuroleptic therapy involves teaching them skills of symptom self-management. This requires training patients to identify early signs of relapse as warning signals and to develop their capability to seek early intervention before full-blown relapse occurs (Wirshing, Eckman, Marder, and Liberman, 1989). For refractory patients who do not respond optimally to somatic and rehabilitative treatments, longer-term placement in an intensive, residential behavior therapy program may yield better ultimate outcomes (Paul and Lentz, 1977).

Rehabilitation Interventions

Rehabilitation strategies improve the patient's independent functioning through acquiring skills and strengthening behavioral repertoires (Wallace and others, 1980). Other rehabilitation strategies compensate for functional deficits by providing social prostheses in the form of case managers, supported employment, residential care homes in the community, or interdisciplinary rehabilitation teams (Liberman, 1987; Stein and Test, 1978; Test, 1984, 1989). Choosing appropriate rehabilitation strategies is based on the assessment of patients' deficits. Thus, lack of social competence, conversational skills, and instrumental role skills should lead to social and life skills training; relationships with family members who are high on expressed emotion and in families in which tension is high and problem solving low should trigger educational and behavioral approaches to family therapy; and lack of occupational skills indicate the need for vocational rehabilitation (Falloon and Liberman, 1983). The remainder of this chapter reviews the manner in which behavioral rehabilitation methods—based on skills training or social support—can be used in community and inpatient settings.

Inpatient Social Learning Programs. For chronic schizophrenic patients with severe deficits that prevent community tenure, an intensive behavior-therapy program, such as a ward-wide token economy and social learning program, may be appropriate. Paul and Lentz (1977) developed and evaluated a comprehensive social learning program for severely disabled schizophrenic patients. This program employed a highly specific token economy and many hours of structured educational activities throughout the day. Patients were positively reinforced with praise and tokens for productive, appropriate behavior (for example, cleaning rooms, attending classes, and grooming) and were fined tokens, ignored, and/or placed in time-out for inappropriate behavior such as yelling or assaulting. They could exchange tokens for back-up reinforcers such as consumables and privileges. Patients were held accountable for their behavior and were provided with training in social skills to equip them for community living.

Paul and Lentz (1977) randomly assigned eighty-four long-term, schizophrenic patients to state hospital units that use social learning, milieu therapy, or traditional custodial care approaches. A multimodal assessment battery, including reliable time-sampled behavioral observations, revealed impressive and clear-cut results favoring the social learning approach. Improved functioning, enabling long-term community tenure, occurred in 97 percent of the social learning patients. The therapeutic milieu program was less effective, but its 71 percent release and community-maintenance rate was still a favorable outcome when compared to the 45 percent rate of patients released from custodial care and living in the community for eighteen months or longer. An important characteristic of the social learning program was that it was clearly the most cost-effective program when decreased need for hospitalization was included in cost calculations.

The apparently outstanding success in sustaining patients in the community was mirrored by significant clinical and behavioral improvements that produced a minority of patients who could not be distinguished from a normal population. After only fourteen weeks of treatment, every resident in the social learning program showed dramatic improvements in overall functioning, regardless of usual prognostic indicators such as duration of hospitalization and pretreatment level of impairment. Moreover, by the end of the second year of programming, fewer than 25 percent of residents in either experimental condition required maintenance psychotropic drugs.

A similar social learning program is located at the Clinical Research Unit (CRU) at Camarillo State Hospital, the longest-running token economy in any residential psychiatric facility. Treatment-refractory and severely impaired patients are referred to the CRU when standard hospital programming proves ineffective. There they are provided with training in personal grooming, social skills, room clean-up, and appropriate meal behavior. Special programs are developed for each patient's unique behavioral problems as well, thus increasing the likelihood of discharge (Liberman, Wallace, Teigen, and Davis, 1974). Most of the patients' days are structured with specific activities and frequent training sessions. Special attention is paid to helping patients learn to pursue recreational activities and other structured activities, and participation in such structured activities has been shown to reduce patients' bizarre behavior (Liberman, Wallace, Teigen, and Davis, 1974; Polsky and McGuire, 1981; Rosen and others, 1981; Wong and others, 1987; Wong and others, 1988).

Behavioral interventions developed at the CRU have been successful in increasing social skills in chronic schizophrenic patients (Massel and others, 1985), in controlling aggressive behavior in treatment-refractory schizophrenic patients and in those with other disorders (Glynn and others, 1987), and in reducing delusional speech among schizophrenic patients (Liberman, Teigen, Patterson, and Baker, 1973). During its eighteen years of operation, 42 percent of the patients referred to the Unit as refractory and requiring more intensive treatment have been discharged into the community, with half of them being successfully maintained in the community for six months to five years after discharge (Banzett, Liberman, Moore, and Marshall, 1984).

Community Support Programs. As illustrated in the decision tree in Figure 1, community support programs are necessary for providing comprehensive rehabilitation services. They can be the locus for skills-building efforts close to patients' natural living and working environments, and are important for maintaining gains made in social skills training, behavioral family therapy, and vocational rehabilitation. Comprehensive rehabilitation strategies must follow patients from the hospital to the community. Skills training modules—comprising training manuals, patient workbooks, and demonstration videos—are an example of a portable and replicable rehabilitation modality that can be used in hospital and community settings, thereby serving as functional bridges for patients moving through the continuum of care (Eckman, Liberman, Phipps, and Blair, 1989).

Community support programs are often as effective as inpatient treatment in reducing symptomatology without increasing the burden on the family or neighbors (Test, 1984). Moreover, patients are often more satisfied with (Polak, 1978; Test and Stein, 1978) and function at greater levels of independence in such programs (Mosher and Menn, 1978; Stein and Test, 1980).

Movement through community programs should depend on incremental skills acquisition and meeting performance criteria such that social functioning ultimately approaches "normal" levels. Although research has shown that as few as three or four training sessions improve interpersonal functioning (Goldstein and others, 1973; Goldsmith and McFall, 1975), Liberman, Nuechterlein, and Wallace (1982) have suggested that several years of training may be necessary to achieve significant impact on long-standing disabled lifestyles. Criteria for placement into more demanding programs should depend on the patient/trainee exhibiting mastery of the skill. Regardless of the duration of training, only when the individual is able to perform the behavior at criterion level in real-life situations can it be assumed that skills are acquired and training is no longer necessary.

Rehabilitation programs rely on (1) educational strategies to improve the patients' skill repertoire and (2) support services to bolster their limited interpersonal network (Anthony and Liberman, 1986). The token economy and social skills training methods used within inpatient settings apply to community social learning programs as well. Social skills training is a generic category whose training techniques are applicable to improving a wide range of interpersonal and instrumental skills (Christoff and Kelly, 1985). The number of skill modules comprising community-based social learning programs is likely to be larger than the available curricula within the hospital. Patients' instrumental and interpersonal goals increase sharply and become more imminent when they move from the hospital to the community. In addition, the community settings available to patients participating in support programs offer greater opportunity for generalization of skills.

Community programs incorporate case management strategies to augment social support networks, link patients with needed services, and advocate for patients' needs. In this way, community support systems assume some responsibility for providing a stress buffer to life events. Test (1979) identified cross-sectional and longitudinal factors that guide case management. In cross-sectional services, case managers ensure that the multitude of agencies available to the patient actually provide the needed community treatment and are coordinated with one another. Longitudinal service describes a continuum of care that follows the patient from community setting to hospital visit and back into the community. In this way, the individual's linkages with community services remain intact (Intagliata, 1982; Witheridge and Dincin, 1985).

Life Skills Training School. First Step, a social learning, community support program located in Evanston, Illinois, is funded by the state's

Department of Mental Health and Developmental Disabilities (Corrigan, Davies-Farmer, and Lome, 1988). It was established as a school for individuals with severe "life problems" to acquire social and coping skills that facilitate community survival. Clinicians were identified as "teachers" and patients were called "students"; the "student" label obviated the anxiety, hostility, and feelings of disempowerment associated with patient status (Katz, 1979). Individuals participated in three 40-minute learning modules daily in a classroom setting, with teachers using social skills training techniques to facilitate acquisition of interpersonal behaviors.

Lazarus divided the realm of human experience into seven domains: Behavior, Affect, Sensation Imagery, Cognition, Interpersonal, and Drugs (health-related behaviors); hence the acronym, BASIC I.D. (Brunell and Young, 1982; Lazarus, 1976). First Step employed Lazarus's BASIC I.D. to organize its broad curriculum; the modules are summarized in Exhibit 1. Assignment to classes was jointly determined by student and teacher based on current symptom level, prior assessment of skill deficits, and learning modules already accomplished. Progress in the class was assessed at the end of three-month instructional periods on a ten-item checklist specific to each learning module. Students who did not meet criteria repeated the learning area the next quarter it was offered.

Bandura (1969) distinguished between the acquisition of skills—through operant and vicarious conditioning—and the subsequent performance of the behaviors. Newly acquired skills may not be performed in the environment in the absence of opportunities to use the skill or in the absence of reinforcement contingent upon displaying the skills. First Step included a token economy to shape newly acquired skills to criterion levels. To facilitate generalization of these skills, token reinforcement was augmented by a step-level system: As the students' level of interpersonal functioning improved, their status, responsibilities, and privileges within the milieu increased. Individuals at higher levels participated in the school government or newspaper, with the highest-level students serving as president or editor, respectively.

To facilitate generalization, First Step included in vivo training in which modules were taught in community settings. For example, the "Community Access" class included riding a bus and navigating a shopping mall. Homework assignments were given and a First Step Club was implemented in one of the residences to assist in carrying out the tasks each evening.

First Step participants received case management from a sister agency sponsored by Evanston Hospital. Case managers identified individuals in the state hospital who met entry requirements and facilitated their release into a community residence. In the community, the case managers played an active role in assuring that patients arrived at school daily and in

Exhibit 1. BASIC I.D. Outline of Skills Training Content Areas in the Life Skills Training School

*B*ehavior

Community Access: Managing public transportation and locating community services

Leisure Training: Introduction to community recreational activities; fun-time scheduling

Money Management: Skills to manage personal finances

Personal Contingency Contracting: Training in self-monitoring and self-reward to attain personal goals (Kanfer and Gaelick, 1986)

Role Playing: For the more severely disabled patient, exercises that desensitize behavior rehearsal.

*A*ffect

Relaxation: A range of relaxation skills varying from autogenic and imaginal exercises to inhibiting anxiety with more active responses (for example, long, vigorous walks).

*S*ensation

Body Awareness: Several exercises to reacquaint the more severely disabled patients with their range of bodily sensations and movements

Hallucination Control: Training in cognitive restructuring and imagery methods to challenge or compartmentalize hallucinations (Rutner and Bugle, 1969).

*I*magery

Imagery Control: Use of imagery for relaxation and behavior rehearsal (Lazarus, 1984).

*C*ognition

Control of Thought Disorder: Identification of stressful situations provoking thought disorder; plan to avoid decision making within these situations

Paying Attention: Operant and self-monitoring techniques to improve attention (Magaro, Johnson, and Boring, 1986)

Rational Thinking: Techniques to identify and counter irrational thoughts (Perris, 1989)

Relapse Prevention: Identifying high-risk situations and creating a plan to avoid relapse (Marlatt and Gordon, 1985).

*I*nterpersonal

Assertiveness: Behaviors that facilitate accomplishing interpersonal, instrumental goals

Conversational Skills: Behaviors including eye contact, body language, and appropriate discussion topics

Family Interactions: Skills to help separation from the family; negotiating skills for family disagreement (Falloon, Boyd, and McGill, 1984)

Pre-Work Skills: Time scheduling; skills to facilitate working with others under supervision

Problem Solving: Problem-identification and solution-generating skills for interpersonal dilemmas (Wallace, 1982)

Sexuality and Dating: How to get a date, birth control, and pregnancy (Lukoff and others, 1986).

*D*rugs

Health: Nutrition and exercise strategies: self-monitoring of physical health

Hygiene: Personal grooming and clothes maintenance

Medication Management: Strategies to facilitate adherence to drug regimens (Liberman, Eckman, and Phipps, 1986).

implementing First Step behavior programs in the patients' residence. Moreover, case managers coordinated treatment with other agencies, advocating for their patients when necessary to make certain that psychiatric, medical, and residential care was adhering to standards.

A two-year, quasi-experimental analysis of the First Step Program was completed (Corrigan, Davies-Farmer, Lightstone, and Stolley, in press). Subjects for this study had at least a three-year history of schizophrenia, multiple hospitalizations, and one to three failures in previous outpatient programs. After eighteen months of treatment, First Step subjects significantly decreased their rate of hospitalization by 82.5 percent. Translated into cost-benefit ratios, the community program was 57.5 percent less expensive than year-round inpatient care and 43.2 percent less expensive than residing in a community residence and receiving only case management. In addition to being measured for rehospitalization rates, subjects in the treatment group were assessed for changes in the acquisition, performance, and generalization of skills (Corrigan, Davies-Farmer, Lightstone, and Stolley, in press). Results showed a steady and significant increase in the acquisition and performance of trained skills. There was evidence that the treatment resulted in generalization of skills to other settings and a broader range of responses, although this trend did not reach statistical significance. The success of the First Step Program replicated earlier demonstrations of the efficacy of social learning methods in community mental health centers (Liberman and Bryan, 1977; Liberman and others, 1982; Liberman and Mueser, 1989).

Summary

Several behavioral rehabilitation strategies have been empirically validated in the treatment of schizophrenia and are now the psychosocial treatments of choice for chronic mental disorders. The stress-vulnerability model and an empirically based decision tree offer clinicians' guidance in prescribing strategies that are particularly relevant for each patient. Hence, behavioral family therapy may be indicated for patients who experience disease exacerbation that results from stressful family interactions. Patients with insufficient social and coping skills may benefit from skills training. Supported employment and job-finding clubs may be indicated for patients with deficits in work skills. The form and programmatic matrix of these strategies differ, depending upon their locus in inpatient and outpatient settings.

References

Anderson, C. M., Reiss, D. J., and Hogarty, G. E. *Schizophrenia and the Family.* New York: Guilford, 1986.

Anthony, W. A., and Liberman, R. P. "The Practice of Psychiatric Rehabilitation: Historical, Conceptual, and Research Base." *Schizophrenia Bulletin,* 1986, *12,* 542-559.

Bandura, A. *Principles of Behavior Modification.* New York: Holt, Rinehart, & Winston, 1969.

Banzett, L. K., Liberman, R. P., Moore, J. W., and Marshall, B. D. "Long-Term Follow-up of the Effects of Behavior Therapy." *Hospital and Community Psychiatry,* 1984, *35,* 277-279.

Birley, J.L.T., and Brown, G. W. "Crisis and Life Changes Preceding the Onset of Acute Schizophrenia." *British Journal of Psychiatry,* 1970, *116,* 327-333.

Broen, W. E. *Schizophrenia: Research and Theory.* New York: Academic Press, 1968.

Brown, G. W., and Birley, J.L.T. "Crisis and Life Changes and the Onset of Schizophrenia." *Journal of Health and Social Behavior,* 1968, *9,* 203-214.

Brown, G. W., Harris, T., and Peto, J. "Life Events and Psychiatric Disorders. Part II: Nature of the Causal Link." *Psychological Medicine,* 1973, *3,* 159-176.

Brunell, L. F., and Young, W. T. *Multimodal Handbook for a Mental Hospital: Designing Specific Treatments for Specific Problems.* New York: Springer, 1982.

Christoff, K. A., and Kelly, J. A. "A Behavioral Approach to Social Skills Training with Psychiatric Patients." In L. L'Abate and M. A. Milan (eds.), *Handbook of Social Skills Training and Research.* New York: Wiley, 1985.

Corrigan, P. W., Davies-Farmer, R. M., and Lome, H. B. "A Curriculum-Based, Psychoeducational Program for the Mentally Ill." *Psychosocial Rehabilitation Journal,* 1988, *12,* 71-73.

Corrigan, P. W., Davies-Farmer, R. M., Lightstone, R., and Stolley, M. R. "An Analysis of the Behavior Components of Psychoeducational Treatment of Persons with Chronic Mental Illness." *Rehabilitation Counseling Bulletin,* in press.

Dawson, M. E., and Nuechterlein, K. H. "Psychophysiological Dysfunctions in the Developmental Course of Schizophrenic Disorders." *Schizophrenia Bulletin,* 1984, *10,* 204-232.

Eckman, T. A., Liberman, R. P., Phipps, C. C., and Blair, K. "Teaching Medication Self-Management to Chronic Schizophrenics." *Journal of Clinical Psychopharmacology,* in press.

Falloon, I.R.H., Boyd, J. L., and McGill, C. W. *Family Care of Schizophrenia.* New York: Guilford, 1984.

Falloon, I.R.H., and Liberman, R. P. "Interactions Between Drug and Psychosocial Therapy in Schizophrenia." *Schizophrenia Bulletin,* 1983, *9,* 44-55.

Gjerde, P. F. "Attention Capacity Dysfunction and Arousal in Schizophrenia." *Psychological Bulletin,* 1983, *93,* 57-72.

Glynn, S., Bowen, L., Marshall, B. D., and Banzette, L. "Compliance with Less Restrictive Aggression Control Procedures." *Hospital and Community Psychiatry,* 1989, *40,* 82-85.

Goldsmith, J. B., and McFall, R. M. "Development and Evaluation of an Interpersonal Skill-Training Program for Psychiatric Inpatients." *Journal of Abnormal Psychology,* 1975, *84,* 51-58.

Goldstein, A. P., Martens, J., Hubben, T., Van Bele, H. A., Schaaf, W., Wiersma, H., and Goedhart, A. "The Use of Modeling to Increase Independent Behavior." *Behavior Research and Therapy,* 1973, *11,* 31-42.

Gottesman, I. I., McGuffin, P., and Farmer, A. E. "Clinical Genetics as Clues to the 'Real' Genetics of Schizophrenia (A Decade of Modest Gains While Playing for Time)." *Schizophrenia Bulletin,* 1987, *13,* 23-48.

Hogarty, G. E., McEvoy, J. P., Munetz, M., DiBarry, A. L., Bartone, P., Cather, R., Cooley, S. J., Ulrich, R. F., Carter, M., and Madonia, M. J. "Dose of Fluphenazine, Familial Expressed Emotion, and Outcome in Schizophrenia." *Archives of General Psychiatry,* 1988, *45,* 797–805.

Intagliata, J. "Improving the Quality of Community Care for the Chronically Mentally Disabled: The Role of Case Management." *Schizophrenia Bulletin,* 1982, *8,* 655–675.

Kahneman, D. *Attention and Effort.* Englewood Cliffs, N.J.: Prentice-Hall, 1973.

Kanfer, F. H., and Gaelick, L. "Self-Management Methods." In F. H. Kanfer and A. P. Goldstein (eds.), *Helping People Change: A Textbook of Methods.* (3d ed.) Elmsford, N.Y.: Pergamon Press, 1986.

Katz, I. "Some Thoughts About the Stigma Notion." *Personality and Social Psychology Bulletin,* 1979, *5,* 447–460.

Koh, S. "Remembering in Schizophrenia." In S. Schwartz (ed.), *Language and Cognition in Schizophrenia.* Hillsdale, N.J.: Erlbaum, 1978.

Lazarus, A. A. *Multimodal Behavior Therapy.* New York: Springer, 1976.

Lazarus, A. A. *In the Mind's Eye.* New York: Guilford, 1984.

Liberman, R. P. *Psychiatric Rehabilitation of Chronic Mental Patients.* Washington, D.C.: American Psychiatric Press, 1987.

Liberman, R. P., and Bryan, E. "Behavior Therapy in a Community Mental Health Center." *American Journal of Psychiatry,* 1977, *134,* 401–406.

Liberman, R. P., Corrigan, P. W., and Schade, M. L. "Drug and Psychosocial Treatment Interactions in Schizophrenia." *International Review Journal of Psychiatry,* in press.

Liberman, R. P., Eckman, T., Kuehnel, T., Rosenstein, J., and Kuehnel, J. "Dissemination of New Behavioral Therapy Programs to Community Mental Health Centers." *American Journal of Psychiatry,* 1982, *139,* 224–226.

Liberman, R. P., Eckman, T., and Phipps, C. C. "Protective Interventions in Schizophrenia: Combined Neuroleptic Drug Therapy and Medication Self-Management Training." Unpublished manuscript, Clinical Research Center, Box A, Camarillo, Calif. 93011, 1986.

Liberman, R. P., Falloon, I.R.H., and Wallace, C. J. "Drug-Psychosocial Interactions in the Treatment of Schizophrenia." In M. Mirabi (ed.), *The Chronically Mentally Ill: Research and Services.* New York: Spectrum, 1984.

Liberman, R. P., and Mueser, K. T. "Psychosocial Therapies for Schizophrenia." In H. I. Kaplan and B. J. Sadock (eds.), *Comprehensive Textbook of Psychiatry.* (5th ed.) Baltimore, Md.: Williams & Wilkins, 1989.

Liberman, R. P., Nuechterlein, K. H., and Wallace, C. J. "Social Skills Training and the Nature of Schizophrenia." In J. P. Curran and P. M. Monti (eds.), *Social Skills Training: A Practical Handbook for Assessment and Treatment.* New York: Guilford Press, 1982.

Liberman, R. P., Teigen, J., Patterson, R., and Baker, V. "Reducing Delusional Speech in Chronic, Paranoid Schizophrenics." *Journal of Applied Behavior Analysis,* 1973, *6,* 57–64.

Liberman, R. P., Wallace, C. J., Teigen, J., and Davis, J. "Behavioral Interventions with Psychotics." In K. S. Calhoun, H. E. Adams, and E. M. Mitchel (eds.), *Innovative Treatment Network in Psychopathology.* New York: Wiley, 1974.

Lukoff, D., Gioia-Hasick, D., Sullivan, G., Golden, J. S., and Nuechterlein, K. H. "Sex Education and Rehabilitation with Schizophrenic Male Outpatients." *Schizophrenia Bulletin,* 1986, *12,* 669–677.

Lukoff, D., Snyder, K., Ventura, J., and Nuechterlein, K. H. "Life Events, Familial

Stress, and Coping in the Developmental Course of Schizophrenia." *Schizophrenia Bulletin,* 1984, *10,* 258–292.

Magaro, P. A., Johnson, M. H., and Boring, R. "Information Processing Approaches to Schizophrenia." In R. E. Ingram (ed.), *Information Processing Approaches to Clinical Psychology.* Orlando, Fla.: Academic Press, 1986.

Marlatt, G. A., and Gordon, J. R. (eds.). *Relapse Prevention.* New York: Guilford, 1985.

Massel, H. K., Bowen, L., Wong, S. E., Mosk, M. D., Zarate, R., and Milan, M. "The Development of a Discrete-Trials Procedure for Training Social Skills to Chronic Schizophrenics: Acquisition and Generalization Effects." Paper presented at the annual meeting of the Association for the Advancement of Behavior Therapy, Houston, Tex., November 1985.

Mosher, L. R., and Menn, A. Z. "Lowered Barriers in the Community: The Soteria Model." In L. I. Stein and M. A. Test (eds.), *Alternatives to Mental Hospital Treatment.* New York: Plenum, 1978.

Nuechterlein, K. H. "Refocusing on Attentional Dysfunctions in Schizophrenia." *Schizophrenia Bulletin,* 1977, *3,* 457–469.

Nuechterlein, K. H., and Dawson, M. E. "A Heuristic Vulnerability/Stress Model of Schizophrenic Episodes." *Schizophrenia Bulletin,* 1984a, *10,* 300–312.

Nuechterlein, K. H., and Dawson, M. E. "Information Processing and Attentional Functioning in the Developmental Course of Schizophrenic Disorders." *Schizophrenia Bulletin,* 1984b, *10,* 160–203.

Paul, G. L., and Lentz, R. J. *Psychosocial Treatment of the Chronic Mental Patient.* Cambridge, Mass.: Harvard University Press, 1977.

Perris, C. *Cognitive Therapy with Schizophrenic Patients.* Elmsford, N.Y.: Pergamon Press, 1989.

Polak, P. R. "A Comprehensive System to Alternatives to Psychiatric Hospitalization." In L. I. Stein and M. A. Test (eds.), *Alternatives to Mental Hospital Treatment.* New York: Plenum, 1978.

Polsky, R. H., and McGuire, M. T. "Social Ethology of Acute Psychiatric Patients: The Influence of Sex, Hospital Environment, and Spatial Proximity." *Journal of Nervous and Mental Disease,* 1981, *169,* 28–36.

Rosen, A. J., Sussman, S., Mueser, K. T., Lyons, J. S., and Davis, J. M. "Behavioral Assessment of Psychiatric Inpatients and Normal Controls Across Different Environmental Contexts." *Journal of Behavioral Assessment,* 1981, *3,* 25–36.

Rutner, I. T., and Bugle, C. "An Experimental Procedure for the Modification of Psychotic Behavior." *Journal of Consulting and Clinical Psychology,* 1969, *33,* 651–653.

Sacuzzo, D. P. "Information Processing Interpretation of Theory and Research in Schizophrenia." In R. E. Ingram (ed.), *Information Processing Approaches to Clinical Psychology.* New York: Academic Press, 1986.

Stein, L. I., and Test, M. A. *Alternatives to Mental Hospital Treatment.* New York: Plenum, 1978.

Stein, L. I., and Test, M. A. "Alternative Mental Hospital Treatment. I: Conceptual Model, Treatment Program, and Clinical Evaluation." *Archives of General Psychiatry,* 1980, *37,* 392–397.

Test, M. A. "Continuity of Care in Community Treatment." In L. I. Stein (ed.), *Community Support Systems for the Long-Term Patient.* New Directions for Mental Health Services, no. 2. San Francisco: Jossey-Bass, 1979.

Test, M. A. "Community Support Programs." In A. S. Bellack (ed.), *Schizophrenia: Treatment, Management, and Rehabilitation.* Orlando, Fla.: Grune & Stratton, 1984.

Test, M. A. "The Training in Community Living Model: Delivering Treatment and Rehabilitation Services Through a Continuous Treatment Team." In R. P. Liberman (ed.), *Rehabilitation of the Psychiatrically Disabled.* New York: Plenum, 1989.

Test, M. A., and Stein, L. I. "Community Treatment of the Chronic Mental Patient: Research Overview." *Schizophrenia Bulletin,* 1978, *4,* 360–364.

Wallace, C. J. "The Social Skills Training Program of the Mental Health Clinical Research Center for the Study of Schizophrenia." In J. P. Curran and P. M. Monti (eds.), *Social Skills Training: A Practical Handbook for Assessment and Treatment.* New York: Guilford Press, 1982.

Wallace, C. J., Nelson, C. J., Liberman, R. P., Aitchison, R. A., Lukoff, D., Elder, J. P., and Ferris, C. "A Review and Critique of Social Skills Training with Schizophrenic Patients." *Schizophrenia Bulletin,* 1980, *6,* 42–63.

Wirshing, W., Eckman, T., Marder, S., and Liberman, R. P. "Management of Risk of Relapse Through Skills Training of Chronic Schizophrenics." In C. Tamminga and C. Schulz (eds.), *Research on Schizophrenia.* New York: Raven Press, 1989.

Witheridge, T. F., and Dincin, J. "The Bridge: An Assertive Outreach Program in an Urban Setting." In L. I. Stein and M. A. Test (eds.), *The Training in Community Living Model: A Decade of Experience.* New Directions for Mental Health Services, no. 26. San Francisco: Jossey-Bass, 1985.

Wong, S. E., Terranova, M. D., Bowen, L., Zarate, R., Massel, H. K., and Liberman, R. P. "Providing Independent Recreational Activities to Reduce Stereotypic Verbalizations in Chronic Schizophrenics." *Journal of Applied Behavior Analysis,* 1987, *20,* 77–81.

Wong, S. E., Wright, J., Terranova, M. D., Bowen, L., Zarate, R., and Zarate, R. "Effects of Structured Ward Activities on Appropriate and Psychotic Behavior of Chronic Psychiatric Patients." *Behavioral Residential Treatment,* 1988, *3,* 41–50.

Zubin, J., and Spring, B. "Vulnerability: A New View of Schizophrenia." *Journal of Abnormal Psychology,* 1977, *86,* 103–126.

Mark L. Schade and Patrick W. Corrigan are research associates at the Camarillo State Hospital/UCLA Clinical Research Center for Schizophrenia and Psychiatric Rehabilitation.

Robert P. Liberman is director of the Clinical Research Center, professor of psychiatry at the UCLA School of Medicine, and chief of Rehabilitation Medicine Services at the Brentwood Division of the West Los Angeles Veteran's Administration Medical Center.

Preliminary evaluation of Ohio's expedited review of claims for the SSI and SSDI disability benefits of mentally impaired claimants supports the efficacy of the program in reducing mean processing time and reducing the use of consultative examinations.

Expedited Social Security Disability Determinations: The Ohio Experience

Cille Kennedy, Rick Tully, Linda Craft, Beth Ullery, Timothy F. Champney, Howard H. Goldman

Social Security disability benefit programs provide the major source of income for millions of severely mentally ill adults across the nation. Participation in these Social Security programs also provides access to medical benefits under the Medicaid and Medicare programs. The decision process for determining who is disabled and thus entitled to receive benefits, and who is not, is inherently complex and understandably time consuming. Yet the cumbersome process—even in the initial stages of applying for the benefits and submitting the required medical evidence to support the claim—is particularly difficult for applicants whose disability is based on mental impairments: severely mentally ill adults. Furthermore, once the application is made, the months spent waiting for a decision about whether or not one will receive monthly cash benefits and medical coverage is a stressful time. Eligibility decisions have a major impact on the lives of severely mentally ill people. Individuals who are denied benefits must find alternative sources of support for themselves and for coverage of their medical and other mental-health-related treatments. Individuals who are awarded the benefits are assured coverage for several years as they work toward recovering and enhancing their abilities.

Portions of this research were supported by grants from The Robert Wood Johnson Foundation and the National Institute of Mental Health.

This chapter describes the Quality Liaison Project undertaken by the Social Security Administration (SSA), the Ohio Department of Mental Health (ODMH), and the Ohio Rehabilitation Services Commission, Bureau of Disability Determination (ORSC-BDD), the state agency under agreement with the SSA to conduct disability determinations for Ohio. The Project was designed primarily to reduce the time between application and decision without compromising the quality of the decision. A brief description of both the SSA's disability benefits programs and the routine disability determination are presented here as a context in which to appreciate the Ohio innovation. Preliminary descriptive data from the ongoing evaluation of the Project are also presented. These data demonstrate the drastic reduction in the time required to process a claim reviewed by the Ohio Rehabilitation Services Commission, Bureau of Disability Determination, as part of the Project as compared to claims reviewed in the routine process.

Disability Under Social Security

The SSA has two disability benefit programs: Social Security Disability Insurance (SSDI) and Supplemental Security Income (SSI). SSDI is an entitlement program for workers of pre-retirement age who are unable to continue working because of their disability. SSI is a needs-based program for those who are poor and either blind, aged, or disabled and who are not eligible for SSDI because of an insufficient work history. The evaluation of disability (described below) for both SSDI claims and SSI applications is conducted using the same procedure and using the same standard and definition of disability. In both programs, the claimant must apply for the benefits and prove that he or she is disabled. The term *disability* for both programs is defined by the Social Security Act and means "the inability to engage in any substantial gainful activity by reason of any medically determinable physical or mental impairment(s) which can be expected to result in death or which has lasted or can be expected to last for a continuous period of no less than 12 months" (Social Security Act, Section 223(d)(1)). The definition of disability refers solely to the ability to work.

Disability Determination

The process by which initial claims for both SSDI and SSI programs are reviewed is called the *disability determination.* The first step occurs at the local level when the claimant goes to the SSA's local district office to file a claim with a claims representative. The claims representative first determines whether or not the claimant is currently working at or above the financial level considered to be "substantial gainful activity" (SGA), and denies claimants who are. For those below SGA, the claims representative decides which program—SSDI, SSI, or both—the claimant is eligible for and forwards the claim to the state's Disability Determination Service (DDS). States have agreements with the SSA to conduct disability determinations.

At the state's Disability Determination Service, a team consisting of a disability analyst and a reviewing medical consultant (a psychiatrist or clinical psychologist for claims based on mental impairments) collects medical information until sufficient evidence has been obtained to make a disability determination. If the team cannot collect sufficient evidence to make a decision—from the applicant's physician, psychiatrist, or other mental health workers—then they obtain a consultative examination in which the claimant is interviewed to provide the additional medical evidence.

Once sufficient evidence is collected to evaluate the impairment, the reviewing medical consultant determines whether the claimant has a severe impairment. If not, the claim is denied based on this medical consideration alone. This conclusion is based on whether or not the claimant's condition results in little or no restriction of activities.

For claimants who are severely impaired, the reviewing medical consultant then decides—based on the medical evidence alone—whether the impairment is severe enough to preclude the ability to work. If so, the claim is allowed. This is known as "meeting (or equalling) the Listings." If this medical determination cannot be made, then the claim continues in the review process.

For severely impaired claimants who cannot be found incapable of work by a medical review alone, both medical and nonmedical factors are taken into consideration. The nonmedical factors are primarily vocational, educational, and age of the claimant. The reviewing medical consultant assesses the amount of residual functioning the claimant has in spite of her or his severe impairment. The disability analyst then combines this medical information with the nonmedical factors to determine whether or not the claimant can do her or his former work. If so, the claim is denied. If not, the disability analyst must determine, given the residual functioning and nonmedical factors, whether or not the claimant can do any work in the national economy. If not, the claim is allowed, and if so, it is denied. Claims that are denied can be appealed.

Quality Liaison Project

The Quality Liaison Project is Ohio's innovation to reduce the amount of time spent reviewing initial claims for disability benefits based on mental impairments. The SSA considers the Quality Liaison Project to be a model and encourages its application in other states. The project has three major aims: (1) to reduce the time between application and the disability decision, (2) to improve the quality of the evidence initially supplied with the application, and (3) to reduce the need and use of consultative examinations. The second and third aims serve to enhance the first. The better the original medical evidence, the less time it takes to collect additional evidence and the fewer consultative examinations are required. Thus, less time is spent before a disability decision can be made. The Project is designed to permit a disability determination to be received by the claimant forty-five days after the date the application is made.

The Quality Liaison Project consists of four major elements: (1) its two unique procedures, the Teleclaim Process and the flagged expedited review; (2) the liaison relationships that have become formalized at the individual, program, and system levels; (3) the training that takes place between the mental health and disability determination systems; and (4) an evaluation and monitoring system that continues to provide feedback concerning the ongoing status of the project in meeting and maintaining its stated goals.

The Quality Liaison Project is currently under way in five cities: Akron, Steubenville, Cincinnati, Columbus, and Toledo. The latter three are demonstration sites of The Robert Wood Johnson Foundation—Housing and Urban Development (RWJF—HUD) Program on Chronic Mental Illness. The Project was conceived in 1984 by the Ohio Department of Mental Health and the Ohio Rehabilitation Services Commission, Bureau of Disability Determination. These two state agencies approached the SSA late in 1986 and began a pilot project in Columbus in 1987. At the local levels, the Project involves the county mental health boards for each of the cities and the district offices of the SSA.

Teleclaim Process. The Teleclaim Process is designed to facilitate the first step in the application process: the claimant files for benefits by submitting the application form and supplies the required medical evidence. This process is conceived to be used when a claimant is simultaneously a client in a mental health agency and has a case manager. In the Teleclaim Process, either the claimant or the claimant's case manager telephones the SSA's claims representative and, over the phone, initiates the disability application. While the claims representative completes the application form, the case manager (and/or claimant) begins to compile the necessary medical and nonmedical evidence. For example, the case manager writes up a description of the claimant's limitations in activities of daily living, social functioning, ability to concentrate on tasks, and degree of either decompensation or deterioration when involved in work-like activities. Limitations rather than abilities are described because a claimant must prove her or his inability to work. Meanwhile, the claimant's psychiatrist or clinical psychologist conducts a mental status examination and supplies a report in order to provide evidence that the claimant has a mental impairment. The limitations in functioning must be a result of the mental impairments.

When the claims representative has completed the application form, it is returned to the case manager and the claimant for signing. After they review it together and the claimant signs the form, it is returned to the claims representative along with the medical and nonmedical information the case manager has collected. At this point, the claim is flagged for easy identification during the remaining process. This completes the Teleclaim Process, which is designed to take eight days when operating properly. The next two days are set aside for the claims representative to receive and review the material and to forward it all with the flag to the Ohio Rehabilitation Services Commission, Bureau of Disability Determination, for the next phase in the disability determination.

Flagged Expedited Review. This review is conducted at the Ohio Rehabilitation Services Commission, Bureau of Disability Determination, by a team specifically designated to handle these reviews. It takes place within fourteen days. The claims are identified by the colored sheets that accompany them (for example, pink for Columbus). The colored "flags" are used to pull the claims from the routine process, and these claims then receive a complete review in an ideal of fourteen days at the Ohio Rehabilitation Services Commission, Bureau of Disability Determination.

In the ideal Quality Liaison Project time frame, the next twenty-one days are set aside for the SSA to complete the payment process. The Project anticipates that most disability decisions will find the claimant disabled and therefore eligible for benefits. The Project is designed to be used by clients of the public mental health system, the majority of whom are considered to be severely mentally ill and therefore entitled to disability benefits.

Quality Liaison System. This system was developed to ensure that effective working relationships are forged vertically and horizontally, across and within the mental health and Social Security systems. The Quality Liaison System is designed for the early identification and resolution of mutual concerns by cross-training the staffs of the different systems and by fostering open communication. When problems emerge, all attempts are made to handle them at the local line level (for example, between case managers and claims representatives). Unresolved problems and system issues are handled at the local administrative level, for example, at the level of the county mental health board. At the state level, the Quality Liaison System periodically reviews the Quality Liaison Project. It also addresses unresolved problems that hold implications for procedural or rule change or that have other legal implications.

Training. Training the staffs of the different systems is a key feature of the Quality Liaison Project. Case Managers, claims representatives, and disability examiners from the Ohio Rehabilitation Services Commission, Bureau of Disability Determination, learn about each other's systems, their respective responsibilities in regard to the claimant/client, and each system's resources and constraints. For example, the mental health case managers learn about the requirements for Social Security disability benefits. They learn about disability determination and the type and amount of medical evidence necessary to support a decision. Claims representatives learn about mental impairments, mental health programs and treatments, and the public mental health systems designed to treat people with severe mental disorders.

Evaluation. Evaluation of the Project is conducted jointly by the Ohio Department of Mental Health, the Ohio Rehabilitation Services Commission, Bureau of Disability Determination, and the National Evaluation team of the Robert Wood Johnson Foundation-HUD Program on Chronic Mental Illness. The sample of claims consists of all Quality Liaison claims, initiated using the Teleclaim Process, in the participating SSA district offices in the five cities listed above, and all other claims, generally self-initiated, that are filed in those same district offices and adjudicated on the basis of a mental impairment. Nonproject claims may include those made by individuals who currently receive services from the public mental health system. Data on the regular (nonproject) claims also include those claimants who are being evaluated on the basis of mental retardation as a primary diagnosis, whereas the data on Project claims do not.

Fifteen months' worth of Project claims data exist for Columbus and Toledo (May 1988 through July 1989); thirteen months' worth for Cincinnati (from July 1988); nine months' worth for Steubenville; and seven months' worth for Akron. In all, 6,995 claims have been reviewed since July 1988 in these sites: 231 Project claims and 6,764 regular claims. Columbus and Toledo account for 86 and 104 of the Project claims, respectively, and 2,221 and 1,494 of the regular claims, respectively. At the other end of the spectrum, Steubenville has processed a total of 6 Project claims and 320 regular claims since the Project began there.

The average number of days from the point at which an application was "teleclaimed" into the district office until the client learned whether or not he or she would receive disability benefits was 46.4 days in Akron, 58.5 days in Cincinnati, 42.8 days in Columbus, 18 days in Steubenville, and 64 days in Toledo. For regular claims, the average number of days ranged from a low of 77.2 in Columbus to a high of 85.6 in Akron. For Project claims, the range was larger: from an average of 18 days' processing time for Steubenville's 6 claims to 64 days for Toledo's 104 Project claims. Clearly, the average number of days varies more for Project claims than for regular claims.

In predicting the average number of days for claims processing over time or as more cities are added to this Project, one might expect the rate to slowly increase as the novelty of the initiative fades. This, however, does not appear to be the case. In the reporting period for May of 1988, Columbus and Toledo averaged 38.2 and 71.6 days, respectively, for their Project claims, and 74.1 and 76.4 days, respectively, for their regular claims. In the July 1989 reporting quarter, Columbus and Toledo averaged 27 days and 50.3 days, respectively, for their Project claims, whereas the regular claims took 71.8 and 72.7 days, respectively.

A major factor in reducing processing time is whether or not the Ohio Rehabilitation Services Commission, Bureau of Disability Determination, needs to obtain a consultative examination (CE) to complete the medical evidentiary requirements for the decision-making process. A consultative examination takes place after the claim has been filed. It is costly to the SSA and time consuming to the client. Obtaining a consultative examination is considered only after the Ohio Rehabilitation Services Commission, Bureau of Disability Determination, has attempted to obtain the needed information from sources who already know the claimant. The determination process is put "on hold" until the consultative examination report arrives.

During the fifteen months for which data are available, 53 percent of the regular claimants were referred for consultative examinations, whereas only 13 percent of Project claimants were referred. The number of claimants referred for consultative examinations varies greatly over time within each of the cities for the Project claims. For example, during one reporting period in Columbus only 4.8 percent of the claimants were referred for consultative examinations, whereas during the following three periods, 23.5, 22.5, and 0 percent were referred.

To date, none of the data have been organized to examine the information gathered on the quality of the medical evidence originally submitted at the time of application. At present, the percent of claims requiring consultative examinations may be viewed as a proxy for the sufficiency of the original medical evidence. One can conclude from the above description that quality of the medical evidence, without obtaining a consultative examination, is sufficient for an average of 87 percent of the Project claims. Sufficient medical evidence is the amount necessary to support a disability decision. Less than half (47 percent) of the regular claims, on the other hand, had sufficient medical evidence without obtaining a consultative examination.

From this purely descriptive exploration of the evaluation data, it appears that the Quality Liaison Project has attained and is maintaining at least two of its three stated goals. The Project has reduced the average number of days between the application for disability benefits and the receipt of a disability determination, although two of the cities do not consistently meet the ideal standard of forty-five days. Nonetheless, the average number of days to reach a disability decision is drastically less for Project claims than for regular ones.

These data offer the cities' Quality Liaison Systems an opportunity to examine the areas in the process that are either problematic or problem-free compared to the ideal. For example, given the seemingly large number of regular claims being filed in comparison to Project claims, each city might review whether that poses an opportunity for outreach or is an appropriate use of the two systems. It may mean that there are individuals who are seeking benefits based on their mental impairments and are not clients of the mental health system. It may also mean that clients of the mental health system do not need or want the special attention of their case managers in this particular application process.

Although no direct examination of data on the quality of the medical evidence was presented, the proxy measure of the need for consultative examinations suggests that the necessary medical evidence could be obtained from sources who knew the Project clients.

In all, preliminary examination of the evaluation data support the Quality Liaison Project and the viability of expedited disability determinations for SSI and SSDI benefits for severely mentally impaired adults.

Cille Kennedy is a staff fellow in the Division of Biometry and Applied Sciences of the National Institute of Mental Health. She is the former associate director of the National Evaluation of The Robert Wood Johnson Foundation—Housing and Urban Development Program on Chronic Mental Illness.

Rick Tully is the assistant deputy director of program support for the Ohio Department of Mental Health.

Linda Craft is the assistant director of operations at the Ohio Rehabilitation Commission, Bureau of Disability Determinations.

Beth Ullery is the chief of programs for the Franklin County Mental Health Board in Columbus, Ohio.

Timothy F. Champney is a research administrator in the Office of Program Evaluation and Research of the Ohio Department of Mental Health.

Howard H. Goldman is director of the Mental Health Policy Studies program at the University of Maryland. He is the principal investigator of the National Evaluation of The Robert Wood Johnson Foundation—Housing and Urban Development Program on Chronic Mental Illness.

The 1985 medical standards and guidelines for the adjudication of mentally impaired claimants for SSI and SSDI disability benefits were evaluated and basically found to reflect the statutory definition of disability according to the current perspective of psychiatry.

The Social Security Disability Evaluation Study

Cille Kennedy, Samuel J. Simmens, Harold Alan Pincus, Howard H. Goldman, Steven S. Sharfstein

In August of 1985, new medical criteria for evaluating claims for Social Security disability benefits became effective for adults whose applications were being assessed on the basis of mental impairments. These new standards and their guidelines apply to disability determinations for both the Supplemental Security Income (SSI) and Social Security Disability Insurance (SSDI) programs. In that year, 1,169,200 claims, based on both physical and mental impairments, were filed for SSDI benefits alone. Of the 377,372 SSDI claims that were awarded benefits, over 20 percent were based on mental impairments. Complementary figures for SSI claims are not available. From these incomplete figures, however, the magnitude of the potential effect of the new criteria on people's lives is evident.

The standards and guidelines were developed by the Social Security Administration (SSA) to reflect current knowledge of the mental health professions. Work groups were convened to include governmental agencies such as the National Institute of Mental Health and professional organizations such as the American Psychiatric Association, American Psychological Association, American Nurses Association, the National Association of Social Workers, and the Mental Health Law Project. Both the standards and their guidelines are bound by the definition of *disability* as stated in the Social Security Act: "Disability is the inability to engage

The authors wish to thank Ernest M. Gruenberg for his valuable contributions to the design and conduct of the research.

in any substantial gainful activity by reason of any medically determinable physical or mental impairment which can be expected to result in death or which has lasted or can be expected to last for a continuous period of no less than 12 months" (Social Security Act, Section 223(d)(1)). Before the new medical standards and guidelines were published, the SSA contracted with the American Psychiatric Association (APA) to conduct an evaluation.

SSA's Medical Standards and Guidelines

The standards and guidelines evaluated by the APA were the 1985 Listings of Mental Impairment (Listings), the Psychiatric Review Technique Form (PRTF), the Mental Residual Functional Capacity Assessment (MRFCA), and the medical evidence requirements. In brief, the Listings, the published regulations, are a classification of mental impairments and resulting functional limitations. Both the Psychiatric Review Technique Form and the Mental Residual Functional Capacity Assessment are forms upon which the assessment of claims is conducted. The Psychiatric Review Technique Form puts the Listings into operation, whereas the Mental Residual Functional Capacity Assessment is applied only to those claims for which a disability decision cannot be reached using the Psychiatric Review Technique Form. Goldman and Runck (1985) describe the Listings; the process of evaluating disability is presented in Chapter Three of that work.

Purpose of the APA Evaluation

The American Psychiatric Association (APA) study was designed to provide an independent, scientific assessment of the medical standards and guidelines, listed above, that would reflect the perspective of current psychiatry, and was bound by the definition of disability in the Social Security Act. The purpose of the study was to evaluate the SSA medical standards and guidelines used in assessing claims for SSI and SSDI disability benefits based on mental impairments. The study evaluated how the medical standards and guidelines operationalized the definition of disability according to current thinking in psychiatry.

In light of the public controversy that led to the creation of the revised criteria, it is important to note what the APA study was *not* designed to assess. The study was not (1) an evaluation of SSA's implementation of the medical standards and guidelines; (2) a comparison of APA and SSA disability decisions; (3) an evaluation of allowance and denial rates; or (4) an *in vivo* assessment of the claimant's ability to work or a face-to-face interview with claimants.

Study Methodology

The study was designed with three components. The first component furnished the bulk of the study's empirical data, and the other two components provided narrative information that was used to interpret the empirical findings of the first component and to develop the recommendations. Our discussion of the study's methods focuses on the first component.

In the first component, seventy-two APA psychiatrists were trained in one of two study conditions. In the first condition, the psychiatrists learned about the legal definition of disability and the Listings and were trained extensively on the sequential evaluation SSA uses, on the Psychiatric Review Technique Form, and on the Mental Residual Functional Capacity Assessment before applying them to training cases. In the other condition, after the psychiatrists received the same introduction to the legal definition, their training consisted of in-depth discussions of the statute and current clinical knowledge as they applied the law immediately to the training cases. This second study condition represented the application of medical expertise to disability decision making with the statute as the standard for disability without interpretive regulations. Although study forms documented the disability decisions in this study condition, they did not guide it as do the Psychiatric Review Technique and Mental Residual Functional Capacity used by the other study condition.

The thirty-six psychiatrists, from five cities across the country assigned to each study condition, were organized into twelve panels of three members each. Each panel was heterogeneous in terms of its professional and demographic characteristics. The panelists in both study conditions were trained to review the claims for benefits and to reach a decision about the claimant's disability status independently, and then convene as a panel. In the panel, the members compared their independent decisions and attempted to reach consensus, although members were not compelled to change their minds against their better clinical judgment merely to obtain consensus.

The sample of study claims consisted of 732 initial claims for benefits that had been recently filed and reviewed by SSA using the 1985 standards. Each claim was reviewed by one panel in each study condition. The claims were stratified by seven of SSA's categories of mental impairments as defined by the Listings (no claims based on substance abuse were included). The categories that were included were: organic mental disorders; schizophrenic, paranoid, and other psychotic disorders; affective disorders; mental retardation and autism; anxiety-related disorders; somatoform disorders; and personality disorders.

In both study conditions, psychiatrists received training on the Clinical Disability Severity Rating (CDSR), which was designed for the study. This rating scale was used to capture the panelists' decisions about the claimant's ability or inability to work at an unskilled job in a competitive workplace environment over the course of customary work weeks. The Clinical Disability Severity Rating is a ten-point scale from -5 to +5 with no zero point. Ratings are made by first deciding whether or not the claimant is able to work. The psychiatrists judged the degree to which the claimant was able to work or not. For example, a +5 meant that a claimant had a low degree of impairment and a high work ability, whereas a +1 indicated some impairment and some work ability. On the other side of the scale, a -5 noted a very high impairment and virtually no work ability, and a -1 was an intermediate degree of impairment and little work ability. Both -1 and +1 are considered marginal ratings in that the claimant is on the border of able/not able to work. At the extreme ends of the scale (+5 and -5), the ability or inability to work is more clear cut. Panelists who used the SSA's standards and guidelines (the Psychiatric Review Technique and Mental Residual Functional Capacity) rated the claimant on the Clinical Disability Severity Rating only after completing the SSA forms. The other panelists filled in the Clinical Disability Severity Rating after their careful review of the case folder. In both study conditions, information was collected about the panelists' confidence in their Clinical Disability Severity Ratings and on their judgment on the quality of the medical evidence contained in the claims.

Briefly, the second study component consisted of a survey of participating psychiatrists' overall reactions to using the standards and guidelines, and a survey of panelists to identify problems they encountered when applying the standards and guidelines to claims. Psychiatrists in the other study condition were queried about difficulties in reaching disability decisions and were asked to suggest potential remediation. In the third study component, a subset of the psychiatrists received additional training on both approaches to disability determination. They then conducted an intensive review using both approaches to adjudicate difficult claims, and they were asked to develop a consensus on the source of difficulty and to develop solutions to the problem.

Study Findings

The general approach to analyzing the empirical data was to compare the panel-level disability judgments of each of the two study conditions using the Clinical Disability Severity Rating. Two statistics were employed: the proportion-of-agreement statistic and the kappa statistic. The proportion-of-agreement statistic was used primarily because it is intuitively understood and can be easily comprehended by the widespread lay and professional audience for the study. The kappa statistic adjusts for agreement between raters (in this instance between panels) that is due purely to chance. The proportion-of-agreement statistic is an inflated measure of true agreement because it includes agreements that are due purely to chance. The proportion of agreement between the two study conditions about the disability status of the claimants was .77. In other words, 77 percent of the time the panel using the Listings, Psychiatric Review Technique, and Mental Residual Functional Capacity, and the panel using clinical expertise and the statutory definition of disability agreed about the disability status of a claimant. This finding was strong enough to substantiate the basic soundness of SSA's revised standards and guidelines.

When applying the kappa statistic to the same data, the agreement between the panels, after eliminating chance agreement, was .46. In the context of the medical literature, this is considered a reasonably good level of agreement for clinical decisions.

The relative strength of the statistics notwithstanding, these summary agreement measures also indicate that there is still a considerable amount of disagreement between the two study conditions. The amount of disagreement attributable to SSA's medical standards and guidelines is important insofar as it permits providing SSA with feedback to enhance the appropriateness and utility of the standards and guidelines. The .23 proportion of disagreement constitutes a data set rich in potential for this purpose.

For those claims about which the panels disagreed, a model was developed to understand the potential source of disagreement. Three sources of discrepancy were identified. The first source of discrepancy is panelist error. Although all attempts were made to double check for this type of error, both through the panel process and the study's quality-control mechanisms, it still must be considered a potential source of discrepancy. The second was that a claim could be inherently difficult. For example, a claimant's ability to work could be truly marginal—a Clinical Disability Severity Rating score of -1 or +1—and similarly trained clinicians might reasonably differ. Another reason for inherent difficulty could be the ambiguity or inadequacy of the evidence leading to opposite interpretations. Finally, the standards and guidelines themselves could be the reason for the discrepant disability judgments of the two panels. Identifying strengths and weaknesses in the standards and guidelines was the thrust of the evaluation effort.

When this model was applied to the study claims, the results were impressive. Using only the psychiatrists' ratings, and without knowing beforehand whether or not the panels agreed or disagreed about a claim, claims were classified into "difficult" and "not difficult" categories.

Assignment to these categories was based on the panelists' ratings of the quality of medical evidence, their confidence in their Clinical Disability Severity Rating score, and the degree to which the Clinical Disability Severity score reflected whether the claimant was a clear-cut or marginal case of ability or inability to work. To control for panelist error as a source of difficulty, only the panel-level Clinical Disability Severity Rating score was used. When the claims were thus categorized, those claims having good ratings on their medical evidence, high confidence ratings, and clear (not marginal) Clinical Disability Severity Rating scores were considered "unambiguous" or "not difficult" claims. Those with poor medical evidence ratings, low confidence in the Clinical Disability Severity Rating scores, and marginal Clinical Disability Severity Rating scores were considered "difficult" or "ambiguous" claims.

In examining only the unambiguous claims, the proportion of agreement between the two study panels rose to .96. The kappa statistic for these same claims rose to .78. These findings endorse the appropriateness and utility of the standards and guidelines as they operationalize the statutory definition of disability in the less ambiguous claims. They also suggest that most of the discrepancy between the two study conditions is attributable to the ambiguities inherent in the claims. In other words, discrepancies are not a result of panel error or problems in the standards and guidelines.

The claims classified as "difficult" provided the pool from which the third-component reviews were conducted. In this review, panelists identified the source of difficulty and developed specific suggestions and methods to resolve the identified problem.

Another approach to understanding strengths and weaknesses in the standards and guidelines was to assess the Listings more directly. One method used by the study was to analyze the data by category of impairment. Claims reviewed under categories of organic, schizophrenic, and anxiety-related disorders all had higher rates of agreement between the two study conditions. Affective disorders, personality disorders, and mental retardation and autism had slightly below-average levels of agreement. On further examination, however, a plausible explanation for the low agreement rate for affective disorders was found: the episodic nature of the disorder itself and the potential inclusion of a heterogeneous assortment of claim types into that category. Finally, somatoform disorders had a low level of agreement between conditions, but the sample size was very small.

The recommendations were developed by combining the analysis of the empirical data with the narrative information gathered in the second study component's survey and the data from the in-depth review of difficult claims in the third component.

Recommendations

The first recommendation was that the basic construct of the SSA's medical standards and guidelines for evaluating mentally impaired claimants should be retained. Second, the standards and guidelines could be improved by making refinements in specific aspects. Taken together, these recommendations offer the opportunity for creative and positive feedback to the SSA. In August of 1990, a regulated sunset clause on the Listings—Psychiatric Review Technique Form and Mental Residual Functional Capacity Assessment—will take effect. The sunset clause will provide a catalyst for making modifications to the 1985 standards and guidelines. For example, the scale points for the fourth functional criterion, which assesses the person's performance in a worklike setting, might be revised.

The third recommendation was that the SSA continue to improve the collection of medical and other evidence. At present, there is no standard national form upon which medical evidence is collected. In Ohio, where an expedited disability review is conducted for claims based on mental impairment, a standard medical evidence form is used with reported satisfaction by the staff.

The fourth recommendation was that SSA consider building upon the study's initiative for the identification and special evaluation of difficult claims. For example, a panel consensus process could be used in assessing claims involving somatoform or personality disorders, which are known to be difficult prior to review. For these known-to-be-difficult cases, SSA and their consultants could develop screening procedures.

Fifth, it was recommended that the SSA consider developing standardized comprehensive training programs and manuals for the clinical staff who review claims. Clinicians receive little or no training about disability in their academic training. SSA should develop more written material to improve the quality of clinician reporting and reduce the chance that SSA would produce idiosyncratic understanding and application of the procedures.

Finally, it was recommended that SSA develop and conduct a systematic series of studies and research development activities related to psychiatric disability in collaboration with academic institutions and professional organizations. One such suggestion was to follow the longitudinal course of the individuals whose claims were so thoroughly reviewed in this evaluation.

Summary

Disability has continued to gain attention as a research topic in the mental health field. Both the SSA and the National Institute of Disability and Rehabilitation Research currently fund research aimed at understanding the vocational needs of severely mentally ill adults, particularly those in supportive employment programs. The National Institute of Mental Health funds research on disability and rehabilitation, particularly research on innovative approaches to increasing the individual's level of functioning and quality of life. All of these federal agencies anticipate continued funding of research on disability. This evaluation of the SSA's 1985 medical standards and guidelines by the APA is an example of the type of disability research that seeks to address issues related to individuals as well as important policy questions. In this evaluation, both the appropriateness and utility of the standards and guidelines were assessed, and the quality of disability decisions for severely mentally impaired applicants was studied.

Reference

Goldman, H. H., and Runck, B. "Social Security Administration Revises Mental Disability Rules." *Hospital and Community Psychiatry,* 1985, *36* (4), 343–345.

Cille Kennedy is a staff fellow in the Division of Biometry and Applied Sciences of the National Institute of Mental Health. She was the director of research and training for the Social Security Disability Evaluation Project.

Samuel J. Simmens is a statistical consultant in Washington, D.C. He was the associate director of research and training for the Social Security Disability Evaluation Project.

Harold Alan Pincus is a deputy director and the director of the Office of Research at the American Psychiatric Association. He was the principal investigator of the Social Security Disability Evaluation Project.

Howard H. Goldman is director of the Mental Health Policy Studies program at the University of Maryland Department of Psychiatry. He was a senior consultant to the Social Security Disability Evaluation Project.

Steven S. Sharfstein is medical director for the Sheppard and Enoch Pratt Hospital. He was the original principal investigator of the Social Security Disability Evaluation Project prior to his position at Sheppard Pratt.

Recent technical advances in psychiatric vocational rehabilitation and related developments have dramatically increased the ability of persons with psychiatric disabilities to attain and maintain competitive employment.

Employment Programming and Psychiatric Disabilities

Robert B. Yankowitz

Three years ago, James Stratoudakis (1986) noted the developing Zeitgeist related to the care and treatment of the chronically mentally ill. Indeed, the 1980s has been a watershed decade during which comprehensive community support, including psychosocial and vocational rehabilitation programs for the chronically mentally ill, has developed into an effective—although still incomplete—system of integrated services. We now have the capability to redress some of the problems spawned in the wake of deinstitutionalization.

This chapter describes recent technical advances in the vocational rehabilitation of persons with psychiatric disabilities, presenting specific examples with empirical results when these are available. It also describes some of the legislative, financial, and organizational developments that have made these exciting advances possible.

Work and Psychiatric Disability

The importance of productive work—whether gainful employment or some other instrumental role performance—as a component of healthy human existence is generally recognized. Including commuting, most of us spend two-thirds to three-quarters of our waking weekdays at work. Besides the obvious economic support and security that most Americans derive from their work, the lucky among us enjoy additional rewards from social relationships, meaningful productivity, and the opportunity for self-fulfillment. The inability to work causes the loss of these concrete and affective benefits. It also results in devastating insult to self-esteem, for work is a principal criterion of normalcy for many people in our society. A survey of 500 chronically mentally ill residents of board and care homes found that lack of work was one of the greatest complaints related to the residents' poor quality of life (Lehman, Ward, and Linn, 1983).

Persons with prolonged and severe mental illness face a host of obstacles unknown to the nonafflicted in the quest for gainful employment. Foremost is the destruction of affective, cognitive, social, and basic task functions, which results directly from the illness. However, the positive symptoms characteristic of psychotic disorders, although incompatible with gainful employment when florid, do not preclude successful work adjustment when in remission. In most cases, these symptoms can be treated adequately with medication, and many patients learn to function successfully with residual positive symptoms through psychoeducation and work-adjustment training. Ultimately more disabling to the vocational functioning of persons with chronic mental illness are the secondary, or deficit, symptoms that are direct sequelae of the illness or that result indirectly from the cumulative effects of insidious functional deterioration and increasing social withdrawal. These include lack of motivation and goal-directedness, hopelessness, avoidant behavior, entrenched fear of failure, difficulty establishing and maintaining social relationships, low self-esteem, poor judgment, poor work habits, poor job-finding and job-keeping skills, and a poor work history.

Lex Frieden, executive director of the National Council on the Handicapped, has said that the most important thing professionals can do for disabled persons is to help them attain employment (1986). Employment is not only a necessary condition for true independent community living with freedom of choice but is the springboard from which persons with chronic mental illness can attain those rewarding aspects of mainstream living that so many of us take for granted: social relationships, family life, entertainment, cultural pursuits, and travel. Yet historically, vocational rehabilitation has been a missing element in the psychiatric rehabilitation system. The majority of our patients attain no employment of any kind; full-time, competitive employment is the rare exception. Although 20 to 25 percent of all persons discharged from psychiatric hospitals are employed at follow-up (Anthony, Buell, Sharratt, and Altoff, 1972; Anthony, Cohen, and Vitalo, 1978; Anthony and Dion, 1986), less than 15 percent of severely psychiatrically disabled persons are competitively employed (Farkas, Rogers, and Thurer, 1987; Tessler and Goldman, 1982; Wasylenki and others, 1985). Despite these discouraging results, psychiatric rehabilitation practitioners have persevered in developing more effective treatment strategies and techniques. Equally as important, administrators and advocates have successfully lobbied to change the structural disincentives that have discouraged the majority of chronically mentally ill persons from seeking gainful employment.

Structural Changes

Historically, services for the mentally ill have never received adequate government support in the United States. Neither the Community Mental Health Centers (CMHC) Act of 1963 nor the CMHC Amendments of 1975 made any provision for psychosocial or vocational rehabilitation. These omissions were caused principally by the political realities of fiscal conservatism and intergovernmental disagreements over fiscal responsibility. During the past ten years, however, complementary forces emerged and began to alleviate this situation. The National Institute of Mental Health's (NIMH) Community Support Program has been catalytic in stimulating and assisting local community support programs and in creating new expectations for rehabilitation and independent community living. The 1978 agreement between NIMH and the Rehabilitation Services Administration establishing two Rehabilitation Research and Training Centers dedicated to psychiatric disability accelerated the development and dissemination of psychiatric rehabilitation technology. A broad-based consumer movement and effective advocacy by interested professional organizations gradually created the political pressure necessary to spark federal legislative initiatives favorable to the mentally ill. Much of this change has had direct impact on psychiatric rehabilitation. Two particular pieces of legislation, Public Laws 99-643 and 99-506, passed in 1986, have had significant impact on the vocational rehabilitation of the chronically mentally ill.

The Employment Opportunities for Disabled Americans Act of 1986 (Public Law 99-643) substantially reduced a major structural obstacle to employment for psychiatrically disabled people: the work disincentives inherent in the federal Supplemental Security Income (SSI) program. Before 1981, a disabled SSI recipient who went to work was subject to a nine-nonconsecutive-month trial work period, at the end of which SSI cash benefits and usually Medicaid were terminated if the recipient was evaluated as capable of earning more than the substantial gainful activity (SGA) level of $300 per month. This occurred even if the individual's total income and resources were within the SSI needs criteria. The work disincentive was clear. Few psychiatrically disabled SSI recipients were capable of earning much more than the SGA cutoff level after taxes and work-related expenses; neither were they likely to obtain a job with health insurance equivalent to Medicaid.

> Thus, only heroic or fool-hardy persons would risk taking a job that did not pay much more than the minimum wage, did not provide

generous health care coverage for pre-existing conditions, and did not offer an immediately secure future with the firm (Noble and Collignon, 1987).

The Employment Opportunities for Disabled Americans Act of 1986 made permanent Section 1619, one of the Social Security Disability Amendments of 1980 designed to create work incentives for disabled SSI recipients. Section 1619(a) provides for special cash benefits to disabled individuals who lose SSI payments because they engage in SGA. In practice, SSI recipients' payments are gradually reduced in proportion to their actual increase in earnings until their earnings reach the break-even point of twice their monthly SSI payments plus an initial income disregard. Under Section 1619(b), Medicaid coverage continues for disabled workers until their earnings reach a much higher level than before 1981. The new law creates additional work incentives for SSI recipients, and recognizes that individuals with severe disabilities often experience discontinuous employment and erratic income. For example, the act extended the period of eligibility during which cash benefits can be restored quickly to a former SSI recipient who has begun to work if he or she becomes disabled again.

The second legislative development to have major impact on the vocational rehabilitation of people with psychiatric disabilities is Public Law 99-506, an amendment to the Rehabilitation Act of 1973. This law created a federal grant program for transitional and supported employment services, and specifically identified the psychiatrically disabled as a target population. It extended the supported employment model first authorized in 1984 for the developmentally disabled (Public Law 98-527) to those disabled by chronic mental illnesses. Supported employment was enthusiastically embraced by practitioners who recognized its potential for vocational rehabilitation with the chronically mentally ill. In combination with the new work incentives of Section 1619 and a low national unemployment rate that creates a demand for unskilled workers, supported employment promises to revolutionize the practice of psychiatric vocational rehabilitation.

Transitional and Supported Employment

Pioneered by Fountain House in New York City in 1957, transitional employment (TE) is an effective and widespread model of vocational rehabilitation for psychiatrically disabled persons. It reverses the traditional vocational rehabilitation approach of "train and place." TE essentially consists of time-limited placement at an entry-level competitive job for a gradually increasing number of hours with on-site support and training (through job coaching), which gradually decreases. The goal is independent competitive employment. TE has been popular in psychiatric rehabilitation because it involves minimal risk to participants, who do not advance to competitive employment until they have clearly demonstrated their readiness. The rapid growth of TE was demonstrated by the Fountain House 1986 telephone survey of facilities operating TE programs (Fountain House, 1987). The survey found increases of 24, 40, and 56 percent in programs, placements, and wages, respectively, over the previous two years.

Supported employment (SE) originally evolved as an alternative to the successful "train and place" model of vocational rehabilitation for the mentally retarded and developmentally disabled. Whereas TE is typically a time-limited entry-level work experience intended to prepare disabled people for relatively unsupported, permanent employment, SE usually consists of permanent employment with a continuous—perhaps permanent—support system built in. Detailed similarities and differences between SE and TE have been described elsewhere (Bond, 1987; Anthony and Blanch, 1987).

SE provides services of unlimited duration required to place and permanently maintain severely disabled individuals in competitive employment (Revell and Arnold, 1984; Wehman and Moon, 1988). In SE, only job development and site preparation are done before an individual is placed on the job. Most services are provided after placement for specific skill training or work adjustment on the job site by a job coach, who may also provide travel training, job analysis, and advocacy (Revell, Wehman, and Arnold, 1984). The transfer of learning required in the traditional train and place approach is eliminated (Vandergoot, 1986). This removes a major impediment for psychiatrically disabled persons, who often have difficulty transferring skills from one situation (training) to another (work). Although the job coach may initially perform a significant portion of the individual's work in order to role model and to satisfy the employer's production requirements (Wehman and Melia, 1985), gradually the coach "fades"; that is, most of the coach's functions are reduced or discontinued as the worker adjusts to the job. Ideally, supportive services remain available continuously and are resumed as needed in order to maintain the work permanently on the job. Permanent employment is the goal.

The SE approach is operationalized in a variety of models, each geared specifically to the needs of particular types of psychiatrically disabled persons. In the *independent placement model,* individuals are placed in totally integrated, competitive jobs in regular business or industrial work sites. The placees, however, receive supportive services as required. In the *enclave model,* four to eight individuals are placed as a segregated work group in a regular business or industrial setting. They receive supportive services, work together in a group, and integrate with nondisabled colleagues during lunch and work breaks. The *mobile crew model* consists of a small group of disabled individuals who, with the assistance of a job coach, perform various types of maintenance work throughout a community. The *affirmative* or *entrepreneurial business* is an independent business operation organized by a rehabilitation agency using disabled employees with on-site support services. The number of variations of the SE model is limited only by the creativity of program developers. The basic concept is simple: develop an employment opportunity to match the functional capability of a disabled worker or workers and then provide training and support services as necessary to maintain permanent employment.

By 1988, twenty-seven states had SE or TE demonstration projects for the chronically mentally ill. It is too early, however, to determine the efficacy of these programs. Since most programs are only a year or two old, too few individuals have been working for adequate lengths of time to draw meaningful conclusions. Two examples, however, are useful to illustrate the potential of SE or TE programs for rehabilitating persons with psychiatric disability.

Eighteen months after its inception, the Schapiro Training and Employment Program (STEP) in Baltimore had already shown encouraging results (D. Shegan, Program Director, Shapiro Training and Employment Program, Baltimore, Md., personal communication, March 1988). Of the ninety-seven chronically mentally ill persons who had been placed by STEP on maintenance, retail, and clerical jobs, 56 percent had worked for six months or longer. Before entering the program, 47 percent of these people had never worked and 63 percent had been SSI recipients. STEP is one of many SE programs operating under the umbrella of the Maryland Supported Employment Project, a successful partnership of state government, rehabilitation agencies, business, and industry.

In 1986, the New York State Office of Mental Health (OMH) initiated its Special Employment Program with start-up grants to fifteen agencies to stimulate the development of innovative vocational rehabilitation programming for the chronically mentally ill. In just three years this OMH initiative has increased nearly sixfold, providing start-up and continuous deficit funding to eighty-five agencies to help support their special employment programs for persons with chronic mental illnesses. These creative and diverse programs include mobile work crews providing groundskeeping and janitorial services, commercial bakeries, restaurants, transitional employment and job placement programs, a microfiche business, and a home health care agency.

Transitional Employment: Case Illustration

The Transitional Employment Program (TEP) at the Mount Sinai Medical Center in New York City started with a small grant from the State

Office of Mental Health and has doubled its client capacity in two years, adding staff through traditional funding sources. In this program, persons with serious and persistent mental illnesses are placed on regular work sites throughout the Medical Center after a diagnostic vocational evaluation and optional period of work adjustment training. They work side by side with regular employees for twenty-five hours a week, and receive job coaching as needed, as well as additional services to prepare them for competitive employment. Participants are placed on competitive jobs with the assistance of a job placement specialist after an average of eight months in the TEP (S. Musante, Program Director, Mount Sinai Medical Center Transitional Employment Program, New York City, personal communication, July 1989). In the two years since TEP's inception in 1987, twenty persons have been placed in competitive employment, including nine with major affective disorders and eight with schizophrenic disorders. Their three-month job retention rate is 80 percent. Of the twelve people who have thus far worked more than six months, only one has been terminated, and three have been working more than one year. Seventeen of the twenty people placed had been tax consumers prior to placement (recipients of SSDI, SSI, or public assistance). All are now taxpayers and have either discontinued consumption of entitlement program revenues or are moving in that direction. In addition, they all enjoy the multitude of benefits usually derived from competitive employment.

The following case illustration demonstrates how several features of transitional and supportive employment enable persons with severe and persistent mental illness to obtain and maintain competitive employment. Mr. A is a 31-year-old black male who has chronic paranoid schizophrenia, borderline intelligence, and severe language difficulties (concept formation and information retrieval). He lacks insight and has poor judgment; he is impulsive, inappropriately talkative, and childishly aggressive with women. His greatest strengths are his personality and motivation. He is very likable and is determined to succeed. Mr. A completed high school in special classes with sixth grade reading and math skills. His sporadic work history as a messenger totaled eighteen months. Before being admitted to Mount Sinai's psychiatric day treatment program, Mr. A had been hospitalized four times in city, state, and voluntary psychiatric hospitals, and had spent almost one year living in the street.

After eighteen months in psychosocial rehabilitation, Mr. A entered the Mount Sinai Rehabilitation Workshop, where he spent five months in vocational evaluation and work adjustment. He then moved to a transitional work site in food service at the Medical Center, where he spent eight months doing porter tasks before obtaining a job with placement assistance in a large food service organization. Mr. A abruptly walked off this job after two days because he was assigned exclusively to pot washing, despite a hiring agreement that he would perform diversified tasks. Fortunately, Mr. A called the program placement specialist, who immediately intervened to arrange his return to work, as originally agreed, to perform porter duties, dishwashing, and simple food preparation. Mr. A has remained very satisfactorily employed for over a year, and lives independently in a supervised apartment. He continues to attend a weekly follow-along work support group and weekly psychiatry clinic medication group.

This case illustrates how numerous elements of supported or transitional employment integrate with other psychiatric services in a successful rehabilitation process. Mr. A first assimilated basic task and social skills through eighteen months of psychosocial rehabilitation to create a foundation for vocational rehabilitation. Eight months of work-adjustment training in the Rehabilitation Workshop enabled him to strengthen the work and interpersonal skills required for job success. These programs were flexible enough to allow him to move through them at his own pace and not start independent competitive employment until he was clearly ready. Job placement services, intervention, and advocacy by Mr. A's job placement specialist enabled him to find and keep an appropriate (selective) job. Ongoing work support and medication groups enable him to maintain stable functioning on the job and in the community.

Two problems needed solving before Mount Sinai's Transitional Employment Program could begin. First, it was necessary to secure the cooperation of Local 1199 of the Drug, Hospital and Health Care Employees Union, since many of the transitional work sites planned were union positions. After the Medical Center's Director of Labor Relations made it clear to the union that the TEP positions were temporary, involved training for people with psychiatric disabilities, and would not replace union employees, the union became supportive of the planned program. Another problem was the source of the wages to be paid to clients while they were on TEP work sites. Almost all Medical Center departments approached to provide a work site were opposed to paying the client wages. Recognizing that clients would need a lot of training and support from site supervisors until they were nearly ready for competitive job placement, the program decided to pay client wages out of its state grant. This decision resulted in a successful and expeditious program launch and an adequate number of work sites with responsive, cooperative, and appreciative Medical Center staff. At least one serious problem remains. There is still no funding source for continuous assisted competitive employment (ACE) services (for example, supportive counseling, intervention, and advocacy), which are necessary to maintain placed clients on their competitive jobs. In New York, the Office of Vocational Rehabilitation funds ACE services, but there are time and amount limitations. These services are not covered by the Medicaid program, and

Community Support Service funds are targeted for other priority groups (for example, the homeless mentally ill). Although many employed clients have coverage for psychiatric services through their employee benefits package, it is usually limited both in amount and types of services. At present, the Mount Sinai TEP and many other supportive or transitional employment programs continue to provide ACE services without reimbursement or direct funding. This practice, however, will eventually cease. As the number of clients needing ACE services continues to grow, programs will be unable to provide it without some form of payment.

The programs in Maryland and New York described above are examples of initiatives occurring nationwide to create a variety of supported and transitional employment programs. These programs may soon provide a data base to demonstrate the cost-benefit efficacy of vocational rehabilitation for the psychiatrically disabled. Although originally developed as federally mandated demonstration projects with state grants, these programs are now achieving permanent status through integration with the traditional service-provider network. Government interagency cooperation at the state level and the establishment of multiple funding streams have been principal factors in this successful transition.

Other Effective Techniques

Post-employment support (PES) services consist of advocacy, case management, and supportive counseling provided after job placement to maintain employment by helping individuals cope with problems that jeopardize job tenure. PES services are a permanent element built into the SE model. They should be available, however, as a highly cost-effective service in all vocational rehabilitation programs for psychiatrically disabled individuals. The logic of expending minimal additional revenue after placement is compelling. Multivariate regression analyses of data from six-month follow-up interviews conducted with 192 former clients of Thresholds, a comprehensive psychiatric rehabilitation facility in Chicago, showed that the only variable significantly related to length of employment was contact with agency caseworker after leaving the agency (Cook, Jusko, and Dincin, 1985). Although this non experimental analysis could not establish causality, it does suggest the importance of PES services to job tenure.

It is unclear at this time what kind of PES services are most effective. Should they be optional, mandatory, individual, group, or some combination? Should PES be conducted in person or by telephone? An elaborate study using an experimental design with random assignment to compare weekly group psychotherapy and additional telephone contact with telephone contact alone found the latter technique more effective in maintaining the job placement of persons with severe psychiatric disabilities (Sands, 1985). PES service is an area that needs exploration through program development and rigorous research.

The *job club* is a low-cost, behaviorally oriented vocational rehabilitation technique shown to be highly effective with nonpsychiatrically disabled populations (Azrin, Flores, and Kaplan, 1975; Azrin and Phillip, 1979). This approach includes classroom instruction in job-finding skills, the provision of professional and material support required in the job-seeking process, peer support, and the expectation that participants commit to the process and take responsibility for finding a job. A modification of the job club incorporating remedial training and a more intensive program structure has been highly effective with psychiatrically disabled individuals (Jacobs and others, 1984). Of the first ninety-seven participants in the program, 56 percent secured employment and 10 percent entered full-time training programs after an average of twenty-four days in the program. Participants who found jobs spent nearly twice as long in the program as those who left the program unemployed. This suggests that job readiness and motivation are important factors in job-finding success. Like post-employment support services, the job club is a successful technique in psychiatric vocational rehabilitation that merits wider application and further research.

Conclusion

The addition of post-employment support services, job club, and transitional and supportive employment to traditional assessment, work adjustment, skill training, and sheltered employment creates a comprehensive array of services adequate for effective vocational rehabilitation across a broad spectrum of the psychiatrically disabled. The growth of effective psychiatric vocational rehabilitation demonstrates the potential benefit of diversified programming for these persons. Yet funding for psychiatric vocational rehabilitation remains inadequate and complex nationwide. Technical advances alone are not enough. What then are the issues we must address to ensure that the long-awaited growth and prosperity of psychiatric vocational rehabilitation does not falter?

Progress has been made in resolving the traditional lack of programmatic responsiveness and financial support from state vocational rehabilitation (VR) agencies for psychiatric vocational rehabilitation. The improved cooperation between VR and state mental health agencies must be sustained and expanded to states that have failed to implement agreements.

There must be adequate financial support within an established delivery system for the chronically mentally ill to benefit from these services. Demonstration projects will wither on the vine without *permanent funding streams.* This requires further structural changes, policy decisions about goals and resource commitments, and increased revenue appropriations or reallocations. Interagency conflicts over responsibility and revenue are wasteful and do not serve clients. Executive leadership and legislative support are necessary at the federal and state levels. Rehabilitation professionals can do more to develop and maintain these supports.

If the necessary financial resources are committed to effective program technologies, there is a real possibility that a significant portion of the chronically mentally ill population can achieve competitive employment, and that an additional portion can attain a meaningful level of vocational activity. The psychiatric rehabilitation community must take the lead in conducting rigorous cost-benefit analyses of the apparently successful programs. The information obtained from these analyses should be an important element in maintaining the momentum of psychiatric vocational rehabilitation.

Finally, we must address the issue of priorities. Should vocational rehabilitation be available for all psychiatrically disabled, or reserved for the highest-functioning persons? Where do we draw the line? The answers ultimately depend on technological innovation, research on and demonstration of cost-benefit outcomes, and the democratic process—the forces that have brought psychiatric vocational rehabilitation this far.

References

Anthony, W. A., and Blanch, A. "Supported Employment for Persons Who Are Psychiatrically Disabled: An Historical and Conceptual Perspective." *Psychosocial Rehabilitation Journal,* 1987, *11,* 5-23.

Anthony, W. A., Buell, G. J., Sharratt, S., and Altoff, M. E. "The Efficacy of Psychiatric Rehabilitation. *Psychological Bulletin,* 1972, *78,* 447-456.

Anthony, W. A., Cohen, M. R., and Vitalo, M. R. "The Measurement of Rehabilitation Outcome." *Schizophrenia Bulletin,* 1978, *4,* 365-383.

Anthony, W. A., and Dion, G. "Psychiatric Rehabilitation: A Rehabilitation Research Review." Washington, D.C.: National Rehabilitation Information Center, 1986.

Azrin, N. H., Flores, T., and Kaplan, S. J. "Job Finding Club: A Group Assisted Program for Obtaining Employment." *Behavior Research and Therapy,* 1975, *13,* 17-27.

Azrin, N. H., and Phillip, R. A. "The Job Club Method for the Job Handicapped: A Comparative Outcome Study." *Rehabilitation Counseling Bulletin,* 1979, *23,* 144-155.

Bond, G. "Supported Work as a Modification of the Transitional Employment Model for Clients with Psychiatric Disability." *Psychosocial Rehabilitation Journal,* 1987, *11,* 55-73.

Cook, J. A., Jusko, R., and Dincin, J. "Predicting Independent Functioning in the Community: Results from a Three-Year Follow-up of Rehabilitation Clientele." Paper presented at the annual meeting of the American Orthopsychiatric Association, Chicago, 1985.

Farkas, M. D., Rogers, E. S., and Thurer, S. "Rehabilitation Outcome of Long-Term Hospital Patients Left Behind by Deinstitutionalization." *Hospital and Community Psychiatry,* 1987, *38,* 864-870.

Fountain House. "Survey Memorandum 287." Fountain House, New York, 1987.
Frieden, L. "Disability Management in the Home and Workplace." Thirteenth Annual Rehabilitation Symposium, New York City, 1986.
Jacobs, H. E., Kardashian, S., Kreinbring, R. K., Ponder, R., and Simpson, A. R. "A Skills-Oriented Model for Facilitating Employment Among Psychiatrically Disabled Persons." *Rehabilitation Counseling Bulletin,* 1984, *28,* 87-96.
Lehman, A. F., Ward, N. C., and Linn, L. S. "Chronic Mental Patients: The Quality of Life Issue." *American Journal of Psychiatry,* 1983, *133,* 796-823.
Noble, J. H., Jr., and Collignon, F. C. "Systems Barriers to Supported Employment for Persons with Chronic Mental Illness." *Psychosocial Rehabilitation Journal,* 1987, *11,* 25-44.
Revell, W. G., and Arnold, S. M. "The Role of the Rehabilitation Counselor in Providing Job-Oriented Services to Severely Handicapped Mentally Retarded Persons." *Journal of Applied Rehabilitation Counseling,* 1984, *15,* 22-27.
Revell, W. G., Wehman, P., and Arnold, S. M. "Supported Work Model of Competitive Employment for Persons with Mental Retardation: Implications for Rehabilitative Services." *Journal of Rehabilitation,* 1984, *50,* 30-38.
Sands, H. "Development and Evaluation of a Psychodynamic Rehabilitation Service Support System Model to Maintain Job Placement of the Ex-Mentally Ill." Postgraduate Center for Mental Health, New York City, 1985.
Stratoudakis, J. P. "Rehabilitation of the Mentally Ill: Psychosocial, Vocational, and Community Support Perspectives." *Annual Review of Rehabilitation,* 1986, *5,* 253-282.
Tessler, R. C., and Goldman, H. H. (eds.). *The Chronically Mentally Ill: Assessing Community Support Systems.* Cambridge, Mass.: Bollinger, 1982.
Vandergoot, D. "Review of Placement Research Literature: Implications for Research and Practice." Washington, D.C.: National Rehabilitation Information Center, National Institute of Disability and Rehabilitative Research, 1986.
Wasylenki, D. A., Georing, P. N., Lancee, W. J., Ballantyne, R., and Farkas, M. "Impact of a Case Manager Program on Psychiatric Aftercare." *Journal of Nervous and Mental Disease,* 1985, *173,* 303-308.
Wehman, P., and Melia, R. "The Job Coach: Function in Transitional and Supported Employment." *American Rehabilitation,* 1985, *11,* 4-7.
Wehman, P., and Moon, M. *Vocational Rehabilitation and Supported Employment.* Baltimore, Md.: Brookes, 1988.

Robert B. Yankowitz is assistant professor of clinical psychiatry, Mount Sinai School of Medicine, and director of psychiatric rehabilitation, Mount Sinai Hospital, New York City.

Traditional approaches to vocational rehabilitation may not always be the best choice for individuals who are challenged ʾoth physically and psychologically. Self-empowerment models ffer a viable alternative and may have applicability across ·fferent conditions.

ultiple Sclerosis Program: Model for Neuropsychiatric isorders

icholas G. LaRocca, Harry L. Hall

. neuropsychiatric condition is any disorder arising from heredity, birth efect, disease, or injury that includes both neurological and psychologial impairment. This chapter focuses primarily on one condition, multiple sclerosis (MS), and on a self-empowerment model to address emıloyment problems in MS. The discussion is presented in the context of comparison of MS and schizophrenia, emphasizing the many experiential similarities between these disorders, how they are subject to many of the same vocational forces, and that a similar self-empowerment model may be effective for both.

The authors mourn the untimely death of Seymour R. Kaplan, M.D., late director of the Rehabilitation Research and Training Center for Psychiatrically Disabled Individuals at Albert Einstein College of Medicine. Dr. Kaplan, whose work spanned both MS and schizophrenia, was among the first to see experiential parallels between the two and first suggested the preparation of this chapter. We also wish to gratefully acknowledge the assistance of Labe C. Scheinberg, M.D., whose persistent commitment to the employment concerns of persons with MS made possible the work described in this chapter.

Preparation of this chapter was supported in part by grants from the Social Security Administration, 13-P-10009-3-01 and 12-D-70287-2-01, the Rehabilitation Services Administration, H128B80070, and the National Institute of Disability and Rehabilitation Research, H133B80018-89 and G0085C3504-89.

Nature of Multiple Sclerosis

Etiology and Pathogenesis. MS is an acquired disease of the brain and spinal cord. Like schizophrenia, the cause of MS is unknown. Many believe MS to be the result of an inherited susceptibility to developing an autoimmune process that is set into motion by the acquisition of an environmental agent such as a virus. Whatever the cause, MS compromises neurological functioning by attacking and destroying the myelin in the brain and spinal cord. Like the insulation in an electric wire, myelin carries no signals but rather makes it possible for the interior of the fiber to do so. When myelin is damaged, the nerves carry their signals more slowly or not at all. Because myelinated fibers are the critical message carriers in all parts of the brain and spinal cord, almost any neurological or intellectual function can be affected.

Epidemiology. MS is similar to schizophrenia in that it is very much a disease of young and middle adulthood. In the United States, the typical age of onset of MS is in the late twenties or early thirties, with the vast majority of new cases (73 percent) occurring between the ages of twenty and fifty. The prevalence of MS in the United States is 58 per 100,000, with an annual incidence of 4.2 per 100,000 (Baum and Rothschild, 1981). Many smaller studies have suggested that the actual prevalence may be much higher, but these claims have never been verified through a national study. Like schizophrenia, the existence of a genetic predisposition is suggested by the finding of higher prevalence in certain ethnic groups (mainly northern European), greater risk in certain families, and by a significantly greater risk in identical twins as compared to fraternal twins (Sadovnick and Baird, 1988; Ebers and others, 1986).

Clinical Aspects. Because MS can destroy myelin in virtually any part of the brain or spinal cord, the list of possible symptoms is long and includes weakness in the legs or arms; reduction or loss of sensation; stiffness; loss of muscle tone; painful muscle spasms; blurred or double vision; lack of coordination of fine movements or intention tremor; bladder, bowel, or sexual disturbances; slurred speech; fatigue; pain; memory loss; word-finding difficulty; impairment in complex reasoning; and many others (Paty and Poser, 1984).

Similar to schizophrenia, MS is notoriously unpredictable and changeable. The typical course is that of slow progression of disability over many years, which can occur gradually or in the form of clearly demarcated attacks or exacerbations. In some cases there is complete or partial recovery from these attacks, whereas in other cases no improvement takes place. MS is thus a disease with extremely wide-ranging effects that are likely to change in largely unpredictable ways. The MS experience takes place in the context of young and middle adulthood when people are in the prime years of family life and career building.

The potential challenges to the individual and family can thus be prodigious.

Parallels Between MS and Schizophrenia

There is no evidence to suggest that MS and schizophrenia share the same etiology. However, on an experiential level they share many similarities that have significant implications for employment. The most detailed comparison of these similarities was published by Stevens (1988). What follows is a brief summary of some of the points covered by Stevens, along with some additional insights.

Stress. It has long been postulated in both MS and schizophrenia that onset and/or attacks may be precipitated by stressful life events. It is difficult to investigate the role of stress in the onset of disease because of the virtual impossibility of following a large enough sample of healthy subjects until a substantial number develop the disease of interest. Thus studies in both MS and schizophrenia have focused mainly on the role of stress in triggering attacks. In MS, more than a dozen studies of stress have been published since 1950. Although early results were largely inconclusive (LaRocca, 1984), recent studies using more rigorous methods have generally found a modest relationship between life events and exacerbations of MS (Franklin and others, 1988; Grant and others, 1989). Much of what was said about MS could be repeated concerning schizophrenia (Rabkin, 1982). However, in contrast to MS, community-wide stressors have been more of a focus in schizophrenia. Stress seems to operate in conjunction with other risk factors for schizophrenia, and as yet we do not understand the mechanism whereby stress may be linked to exacerbations of mental illness (Dohrenwend and Egri, 1981).

Epidemiology. Schizophrenia is more prevalent than MS: at least 600 per 100,000 in North America (Dohrenwend and others, 1980) as opposed to 60 per 100,000 for MS (Baum and Rothschild, 1981). Although not inherited directly as is Huntington's Disease, both MS and schizophrenia appear to have a strong genetic component. Familial concordance rates are similar. The concordance rates for monozygotic twins are approximately 40 to 50 percent in MS (Ebers and others, 1986) and approximately 50 to 60 percent in schizophrenia (Stevens, 1988). In contrast, both disorders show a concordance rate among dizygotic twins that is approximately the same as that among siblings: 5 to 10 percent. Thus MS and schizophrenia appear to be the result of both genetic and environmental determinants.

Pathological Changes in the Brain. MS is accompanied by a number of changes in the brain and spinal cord, including sclerotic plaques at the site of demyelinative lesions, and, in some cases, enlargement of the ventricles and cerebral atrophy. Except for sclerotic plaques, similar changes have been observed in schizophrenia (Stevens, 1988). Since many of these pathological changes may be associated with impaired brain functioning, the issue of cognitive dysfunction cannot be overlooked in MS and schizophrenia (Rao, 1986; Bilder, Mukherjee, Rieder, and Pandurangi, 1985), especially if they compromise functioning in work or family roles.

Onset and Course. Although schizophrenia generally has its onset earlier than MS, both are diseases that first manifest symptoms in young adulthood (Baum and Rothschild, 1981; Stevens, 1988). Since MS and schizophrenia disrupt life just when people are in the midst of education, career, and family formation, their appearance often signals an abrupt change or reversal of life patterns. Following onset, the course of MS and schizophrenia share many features (Stevens, 1988). In both, there may be only a single attack with complete recovery, though this is not likely. In general, the course is characterized by a slowly progressive increase in impairment. In some cases there are clearly defined attacks leading to greater impairment. These attacks may be followed by a partial or complete remission of symptoms, although in some instances there is no remission at all. In other cases, progression is slow and insidious without definite attacks. Although the course of MS and schizophrenia can be described in general terms, in individual cases it is difficult to predict the frequency of attacks, how severe they will be, and the degree of recovery that will take place.

These sobering facts constitute what is perhaps the single most significant issue in employment for both MS and schizophrenia. In both cases, even if there is recovery from an attack and work can be resumed, there is always a sense of uncertainty about the future. An attack may occur at any time, making work difficult or impossible. Thus it is not surprising that persons with MS or schizophrenia, once they have qualified for SSDI benefits, may be reluctant to give them up and go back to work, knowing that at any time, perhaps five years from now, they may have an attack and need those benefits again. It is these very issues that the MS Intervention Model was designed to address and that make such a model applicable in many similar disorders.

Impact of MS on Employment

Through a number of surveys, much is known about employment in MS (Kornblith, LaRocca, and Baum, 1986; LaRocca, Kalb, Scheinberg, and Kendall, 1985; Bauer, Firnhaber, and Winkler, 1965; Scheinberg and others, 1980). More than 90 percent of persons with MS have a work history, and approximately 60 percent were working at the onset of their disease. However, this percentage declines over the course of the illness, and, on the average, only about 25 percent of persons with MS are employed.

Although greater physical impairment reduces the likelihood that someone with MS will be working, the physical aspects of MS do not come close to fully explaining the high rate of unemployment (Kornblith, LaRocca, and Baum, 1986; LaRocca, Kalb, Scheinberg, and Kendall, 1985).

Relatively little is known concerning the specifics of how MS affects employment. Kornblith, LaRocca, and Baum (1986) have described some of these factors. Although mobility problems are clearly a major factor, many other forces are also at work. For example, women with MS are less likely to be working, especially if they are married. Lower educational level also increases the likelihood of being unemployed, especially for men. Recent findings suggest that the presence of cognitive dysfunction is related to unemployment, independent of physical disability and duration of illness (Rao, 1989). Other factors that are predictive of unemployment include symptoms of fatigue, the presence of a spouse who is working, and higher family incomes (Genevie, Kallos, and Struening, 1987).

The picture for schizophrenia is no less complex but is perhaps a bit more problematic. Employment rates for former psychiatric patients tend to be around 10 to 20 percent (Anthony and Nemec, 1983). Former patients more likely to be employed include those who are female, younger, better educated, married, and those who have a more extensive work history and less severe illness (Carpenter and Black, 1986). In contrast to the relatively well-educated person with MS who generally has a work history, the schizophrenic referred for vocational rehabilitation is likely to have little education and no work history (Black, 1977). Both are likely to be experiencing restriction in social and leisure activities, though for different reasons. For the person with schizophrenia, impaired social skills may present a significant challenge to success on the job. Both may have cognitive problems that interfere with learning, planning, and judgment. Moreover, both are subject to the challenges inherent in stigma and in being "different."

Employment Initiatives for Persons with Disabilities

A Host of Alternatives. Until recently, there were no employment initiatives specifically designed for MS. Rather, persons with MS had to take their chances along with anyone else in programs designed to serve multiple populations.

Before the introduction of drugs to control the psychotic symptoms of schizophrenia, there was little impetus for or possibility of vocational rehabilitation with the chronically mentally ill. It was not until the 1950s that mental illness was included among the conditions that could be served by state VR agencies (Black, 1988). In 1978, a memorandum of understanding was signed by the National Institute of Mental Health and the Rehabilitation Services Administration (Black and Kase, 1986). This agreement encouraged state agencies responsible for mental health services and vocational rehabilitation to develop joint programs.

The largest single governmental employment initiative is the *federal/state system of vocational rehabilitation agencies.* Following evaluation, each client may go through a period of individual counseling, training, education, or a combination of these. When the individual is considered job-ready, a placement counselor may become involved. During this process, the individual may be referred to a sheltered workshop or other specialized employment service. In short, the VR agency acts as a sort of coordinating point for assessment and rehabilitation services.

One of the oldest forms of employment service is the *sheltered workshop.* This alternative permits disabled individuals to work for pay outside the milieu of competitive employment. However, there is little record of these workshops employing many persons with MS, and those with mental illness were often rejected. The first sheltered workshop in the United States specifically designed for mental illness was that of Altro Work Shops in the Bronx (Bellak, Black, Abraham, and Miller, 1956). Since that time, sheltered workshops for the mentally ill have flourished both on the grounds of large state hospitals and, with increasing deinstitutionalization, in community-based centers. Sheltered workshops have never been popular with persons who have MS. Sheltered work is often low-level physical work, and since the typical person with MS has a white collar work history, a solid education, but impaired physical abilities, sheltered workshops are generally a poor choice. Moreover, for both groups, the sheltered workshop represents a segregated form of employment with the potential for increasing the sense of being "different" and "dependent."

The *supported work* concept attempts to bring a bit of the "shelter" of sheltered workshops into regular, competitive work settings. Supported work generally includes some sort of training or preparation in job-related skills, preferably on the job; the services of a "job coach" who provides consultation, supervision, and liaison with the employer; case management to coordinate services; and long-term follow-up (Federal Register, 1984). The concept of supported work is a relatively recent one, so results are difficult to evaluate.

Transitional work for persons with psychiatric disabilities was pioneered by Fountain House in New York City (Black, 1988). The typical arrangement entails an agreement between some agency and an employer to set aside one or more entry-level positions that can be filled on a temporary basis by clients of the agency. The goal is to use the position to train clients for entry into the competitive employment arena. No similar programs have been implemented in MS, although the concept of transitional work is often used. Persons with MS who seek to return to work are often placed in temporary and/or unpaid positions to assist them in getting used to working again.

Entrepreneurial models have in part evolved out of sheltered workshops (Black, 1988). In recent years a number of such businesses have sprung up, and, in contrast to sheltered workshops, compete in the open marketplace, pay going wage rates, and operate at a profit. Such businesses run the gamut from Los Angeles's "Corporate Cookie," a gourmet cookie shop run by ex mental patients, to New York's "Binding Together," a printing and duplication shop run by homeless individuals. There are no such programs specifically targeted toward MS, and they would appear to have had little or no impact at present on the employment problems of the person with MS.

The *projects with industry* (PWI) model has been one of the most successful in recent years and serves as the basis for the MS Intervention Model. The underlying concept of the projects with industry is to increase collaboration between private industry and rehabilitation agencies (Black, 1988). Implementation of the model varies, with some PWIs emphasizing job placement or networking with job-ready clients, whereas others incorporate on- or off-site training to prepare clients for jobs. Many focus on a particular industry, an industry association, or a labor union. Although many projects with industry programs overlap with more traditional approaches, the projects with industry tend to emphasize networking and placement in competitive employment and de-emphasize lengthy evaluation, counseling, and off-site training. Many in the MS field who had disappointing experiences with other models began to explore the projects with industry model in the early 1980s. The projects with industry model has been applied in both MS and psychiatric disabilities with a record of approximately 50 percent placement in competitive employment (National Association of Rehabilitation Facilities, 1986).

State VR's Handling of MS. State VR agencies report data through the RSA-300 system. Analyses of the experience of persons with MS and of those with psychiatric disabilities have been undertaken in collaborative projects between Columbia University and Albert Einstein College of Medicine (Kallos, Genevie, Struening, and Andrews, 1988). The federal/state VR system was generally in a period of retrenchment during the years between 1978 and 1984. Referrals dropped 35 percent and total rehabilitants dropped 13 percent. MS appears to have run counter to this trend to some extent. MS referrals were only down 14 percent, and total rehabilitants actually increased by 9 percent. However, the trend was downward for successful rehabilitation of MS clients accepted as eligible for services, declining from 54 percent in 1978 to 51 percent in 1984. These rates continued to lag behind those reported for other physical disabilities: 66 percent for 1978 and 62 percent for 1984. The figures are even more startling when one considers that many of those "rehabilitated" did not go into competitive employment but were rehabilitated as "independent homemakers." In 1984, for example, there were a total of only 806 MS rehabilitants reported by all 50 states, Puerto Rico, and the District of Columbia—an average of little more than 15 per state.

The trend was also down during the 1978 to 1984 period for psychotic disorders, with referrals dropping 36 percent and the total number rehabilitated falling 8 percent. The proportion of clients accepted for services who were rehabilitated remained low but did show some improvement, moving from 43 percent in 1978 to 49 percent in 1984.

The Job-Raising Program. Dissatisfaction with the results of existing programs led many in the MS field to search for alternatives. One such effort, the MS Back-to-Work Training Program (later called Operation Job Match), was funded in 1980 by the Rehabilitation Services Administration as a demonstration project. The program was run by the National Capitol Chapter of the National Multiple Sclerosis Society in Washington, D.C. The MS Back-to-Work Program sought to match persons who had MS with jobs identified through a network of corporate and small business sponsors, forming an MS Job Bank. To prepare people for these positions, the program had a series of structured, educationally oriented group meetings where topics such as interviewing skills and job-related stress were covered. Peer helpers were used extensively in these meetings. The program was successful, and interest developed in replicating the program in other areas.

For several years the Research and Training Center for MS at Albert Einstein College of Medicine (RTCMS) experimented with a variety of approaches to vocational rehabilitation in MS with support from the Rehabilitation Services Administration (Scheinberg and others, 1980; Scheinberg, 1978; Scheinberg, 1980). These efforts included training sessions by RTCMS staff for counselors at VR offices, placement of a part-time state VR counselor in the RTCMS clinic, and establishment of a comprehensive pre-vocational workshop at the clinic. None of these initiatives produced satisfactory results, so it was decided to try a totally different approach. With funding from RSA, a project with industry was set up in September, 1983. This project was a collaborative effort of Einstein, The Development Team, Inc., and the National MS Society. It drew upon the experience of the MS Back-to-Work Program, but with a number of new elements, including expansion to several sites throughout the United States.

The Job-Raising program has many elements applicable to psychiatric rehabilitation, although it was originally designed for MS clients. Job-Raising sites are generally local National Multiple Sclerosis Society chapters. Participants may be unemployed and looking for work, employed and trying to keep their jobs, or employed and desirous of changing jobs. The program consists of ten structured group meetings, with eight to ten participants, in which the focus is on job readiness and job-seeking skills. Following this set of meetings, many sites also have a participant-run job club in which members engage in a job-search meeting for networking and mutual support of their efforts. There are no "placement" specialists. It is an assumption of the program that following brief group training, most individuals are fully capable of finding jobs on their own, often with networking assistance from business volunteers and other job seekers.

More than 1,800 persons with MS have entered the program in more than two dozen sites throughout the United States. All participants are followed for a two-year period following entry, and are considered successful if they retain their job or get a new job and work for at least sixty days during the two-year follow-up period. To date, approximately half have completed the two-year follow-up period. Of those who were seeking new jobs, approximately half have been successful.

Among the unemployed who have entered the Job-Raising program, approximately one-fifth were SSDI recipients at the time of entry. Thus far, the SSDI recipients have been less successful than the rest of the participants in returning to work. Of those completing the two-year follow-up period, less than one-third of the SSDI recipients have been successful compared to more than half of the nonrecipients. This discrepancy led the development team to search for explanations and for ways to better address the employment needs of SSDI recipients. Informal discussion with Job-Raising participants on SSDI revealed them to be less concerned over the loss of benefits if they returned to work and more concerned about the potential difficulty in getting benefits reinstated should they return to work for a few years and then experience an exacerbation.

Where reinstatement is concerned, persons with MS face the same dilemma as many other SSDI recipients who have a relapsing/remitting condition such as schizophrenia, major depression, or arthritis. The process of qualifying for SSDI or SSI can be a long and arduous one. Having once surmounted the seemingly insurmountable and knowing that their disease may worsen at any time, Job-Raising participants on SSDI may be reluctant to risk going through the process a second time with an uncertain outcome. Another disincentive centers on medical insurance. Job-Raising participants might be willing to trade their SSDI benefits for wages but are concerned about the eventual loss of Medicare and the very real possibility that a private insurer in their new job will refuse to cover them. The MS Intervention Model was conceived to address these and other concerns. Although targeted toward an MS population, its basic elements are applicable to almost any relapsing/remitting disorder.

MS Intervention Model

The MS Intervention Model seeks to assist SSDI recipients who have MS to return to work using a two-pronged approach, which addresses many of the same problems and issues that haunt psychiatric rehabilitation. First, the program provides a specialized set of employment services. Second, successful participation in the program qualifies participants for an improved work incentive consisting of a waiver of parts of the law governing SSDI.

Funding and Administrative Structure. The MS Intervention Model (MSIM) is funded under the Social Security Administration's Research Demonstration Program. It began operations in October, 1987 under the auspices of The Development Team, Inc. (TDTI) of Arlington, Virginia. The program was designed to involve 100 individuals with MS who are unemployed and receiving SSDI. Approximately nine sites will participate, all involving chapters of the National Multiple Sclerosis Society and, in some cases, other organizations as well. In each site, local staff are responsible for day-to-day operation of the program following training by TDTI. Staff at TDTI provide ongoing supervision of local sites and consultation when needed. Data are collected in each site concerning participants and their progress through the program and then fed to a central computer data bank at TDTI.

Goals of the Program. The goal of the program is to assist SSDI recipients who have MS to return to competitive employment and continue working as long as possible. The program attempts to accomplish these goals through a specialized set of employment services. The rationale for and characteristics of each component are described below.

Intensive Outreach/Marketing. It is assumed that only through aggressive outreach and marketing is it possible to help substantial numbers of potential participants seriously consider the program. The primary mechanism is a series of direct mailings to persons with MS residing within the geographic target area of each site. Two mailing lists are used. First, the Social Security Administration (SSA) provides a list of names and addresses of all SSDI recipients who have MS living in a given area. Each grantee who receives such information must agree to a set of assurances protecting the confidentiality of these data. In addition to the SSA lists, outreach is also accomplished through NMSS membership lists.

Each mailing includes a brochure describing the program along with a postpaid reply card. Persons returning the postcard are contacted by phone by project staff and are screened to determine whether they are appropriate for the program. In each site, approximately twelve participants are selected and invited to attend the group training program.

Screening and Referral to State VR. Screening may reveal that an individual is not eligible for the program or that he or she needs other services prior to or beyond the scope of the program. In some instances, a referral to the state VR agency could prove helpful. Such a referral can be in addition to or in lieu of participation in the MS Intervention Model. In the majority of cases there is a referral to VR at some point.

Structured Short-Term Group Training. An important part of the program is a series of twelve weekly structured group sessions lasting approximately 2½ to 3 hours each and involving eight to twelve participants and a facilitator. The meetings use a combination of didactic and peer-interaction approaches to cover a variety of topics and issues. Major topics covered include employment objectives, résumé preparation, job hunting, interviewing, negotiating, stress management, assertiveness, communication, planning, pacing workloads, and social relations in the workplace. In addition, because SSDI recipients who have MS have often been out of work and receiving benefits for some time, the groups are designed to deal with issues such as dependency, self-image, anger, fear of rejection, and distrust of "the system." This part of the program is modeled largely on the approach used in the Job-Raising program. In particular, emphasis is placed on a self-empowerment model in order to counteract the dependency-oriented nature of the medical and bureaucratic models that participants may have had to deal with in the past.

Job-Search Services. Following the group experience, each participant engages in an individualized job search with assistance from program staff and participants. Since there are no placement counselors, participants must assume responsibility for "placing" themselves in jobs. Staff and participants assist in formulating employment objectives during the group sessions. Once the job search begins, consultation, assistance, and supportive contact is available, often from a volunteer in the business community. These are also available through a Job Club, a self-help group that forms as an extension of the structured group. In the Job Club, participants compare notes concerning their job-hunting experiences, trade advice and hints, exchange information concerning contacts and prospects, and generally provide emotional support and confidence building during this challenging period of expectation and frustration. Through the Job Club, the process of networking can get off to a vigorous start.

The concept of a Job-Finding Club was first described by Nathan Azrin (Azrin, Flores, and Kaplan, 1975) and has been highly successful with clients who have developmental and psychiatric disabilities. Such programs generally use a combination of peer-group support, counseling, and specific feedback to facilitate the job-hunting process. The emphasis, though, is on an independent and self-directed search. This model shares many of the characteristics of the MS intervention model.

Follow-up. At times, job hunting does not meet with immediate success. For this reason, the program maintains contact with all participants for two years following entry. Follow-up has two major goals. First, it allows program staff to offer a certain amount of emotional support and encouragement during what may be a long and arduous period. Second, it provides a mechanism to track program results and to document qualification for the special waiver. Participants thus have a stake in the follow-up process since it is the mechanism for verifying their right to receive the waiver.

Improved Work Incentives. As mentioned above, many of the employment services offered by this program had already been tried in the Job-Raising program. They met with only limited success for SSDI recipients. Although some programmatic elements have been added to better address the needs of the SSDI target group, the real difference is in the availability of a special work incentive. "Work incentives" are provisions in the SSA regulations designed to encourage recipients to return to work by providing a variety of cushions and buffers to protect recipients against abrupt and/or permanent loss of benefits. For instance, there is a trial work period permitting recipients to work and still receive SSDI benefits for nine months plus a three-month grace period. Medicare continues during this time and for another three years after that. There is also an "extended period of eligibility" that generally begins the month after the end of the trial work period and extends for three years. During these three years, if the individual stops work, benefits can be started again by notifying SSA. No new application, evaluation of disability, or waiting period is needed. Moreover, Medicare benefits continue during this three-year period and for at least three months thereafter (Social Security Administration, 1988). This provision is especially important because it helps remove the fear of returning to work and never being able to qualify for benefits again—a terrifying prospect for anyone with a relapsing/remitting illness. If disability were fixed and stable, the individual could have reasonable confidence that the nine-month trial work period would indicate whether or not he or she could continue working for the foreseeable future. However, someone with a relapsing/remitting disorder can have no such assurances.

A major rationale of this demonstration project was that SSDI recipients need *both* specialized employment services and enhanced work incentives if they are to return to work in substantial numbers. SSA agreed and has granted to qualified project participants a special work incentive consisting of a waiver of the law governing the extended period of eligibility and Medicare. This waiver is granted to anyone who meets all of the following conditions: (1) qualifies for the program, (2) finishes the training, (3) is verified as employed for at least sixty days above the minimum for substantial gainful activity ($500 as of 1/1/90), and (4) completes the nine-month trial work period within two years following verification of sixty days of employment above SGA. Individuals who so qualify are entitled to an extended period of eligibility lasting thirteen years rather than the normal three years. In addition, Medicare coverage will continue throughout the thirteen years. This special work incentive serves two purposes: first, it is designed to provide an incentive for people to enter the program, and second, it is designed to help remove some of the fear of returning to work and eventually relinquishing eligibility for SSDI and Medicare.

Implications for Psychiatric Rehabilitation

We hope this chapter has convinced you that all who live with an unpredictable, incurable, relapsing/remitting disorder have much in common. A major theme has been that this commonality extends particularly to the arena of employment issues.

Employment Service Programs. Employment services will not be effective if they do not reach the target population. Moreover, the target population is not likely to simply walk in and ask for them. Intensive outreach/marketing that presents the services in an attractive and encouraging light is essential. Self-empowerment is probably best encouraged in a peer-group setting. This may be particularly true for individuals accustomed to dependency-encouraging and authoritarian treatment models. The peer group provides an ideal setting for mutual support and social networking. In addition, such groups should have a didactic component and a clear objective. There are many easily acquired skills that can make a big difference in job hunting. The goal should be to help people take charge of and manage their future employment. Thus, even after the formal part of the program is ended, a more informal job club may assist with continued networking and social support during the job search.

Role of Work Incentives. There is considerable fear, confusion, and distrust of "the system." Employment service programs are not likely to be effective if they ignore the reality of perceived disincentives and focus exclusively on the delivery of services. The uncertainty inherent in any relapsing/remitting illness mandates caution if one is considering trading hard-won benefits for an unpredictable stint of work and even less reliable health insurance.

Self-Empowerment Model. Where psychiatric rehabilitation is concerned, probably no part of the MS Intervention Model is more applicable than the concept of self-empowerment. Perhaps our well-intentioned attempts to "evaluate," "train," "counsel," and "place" the unemployed are misdirected. What we may need to do instead is to help persons with disabilities to set themselves free—free to discover and implement the potentialities that were always present but that have been clouded and suppressed by illness and the dependency that even the most well-intentioned caregivers may inadvertently encourage.

References

Anthony, W. A., and Nemec, P. "Rehabilitation." In A. S. Bellack (ed.), *Treatment and Care for Schizophrenia.* New York: Grune & Stratton, 1983.

Azrin, N., Flores, T., and Kaplan, S. "Job-Finding Club: A Group-Assisted Program for Obtaining Employment." *Behavior Research and Therapy,* 1975, *13,* 17-27.

Bauer, H. J., Firnhaber, W., and Winkler, W. "Prognostic Criteria in Multiple Sclerosis." *Annals of the New York Academy of Sciences,* 1965, *122,* 542-551.

Baum, H. M., and Rothschild, B. B. "The Incidence and Prevalence of Reported Multiple Sclerosis." *Annals of Neurology,* 1981, *10,* 420-428.

Bellak, L., Black, B. J., Abraham, L., and Miller, J. A. "Rehabilitation of the Mentally Ill Through Controlled Transitional Employment." *American Journal of Orthopsychiatry,* 1956, *26,* 285-292.

Bilder, R. M., Mukherjee, M., Rieder, R. O., and Pandurangi, A. K. "Symptomatic and Neuropsychological Components of Defect States." *Schizophrenia Bulletin,* 1985, *11,* 409-419.

Black, B. J. "Substitute Permanent Employment for the Deinstitutionalized Mentally Ill." *Journal of Rehabilitation,* 1977, *43,* 5-6.

Black, B. J. *Work and Mental Illness: Transitions to Employment.* Baltimore, Md.: Johns Hopkins University Press, 1988.

Black, B. J., and Kase, H. M. "Changes in Programs over Two Decades." In B. J. Black (ed.), *Work as Therapy and Rehabilitation for the Mentally Ill.* New York: Altro Health and Rehabilitation Services, 1986.

Carpenter, M. D., and Black, B. J. "Review of Research and Evaluation." In B. J. Black (ed.), *Work as Therapy and Rehabilitation for the Mentally Ill.* New York: Altro Health and Rehabilitation Services, 1986.

Dohrenwend, B. P., Dohrenwend, B. S., Gould, M. S., Link, B., Neugebauer, R., and Wunsch-Hitzig, R. *Mental Illness in the United States: Epidemiological Estimates.* New York: Praeger, 1980.

Dohrenwend, B. P., and Egri, G. "Recent Stressful Life Events and Episodes of Schizophrenia." *Schizophrenia Bulletin,* 1981, *7,* 12-23.

Ebers, G. C., Bulman, D. E., Sadovnick, A. D., Paty, D. W., Warren, S., Hader, W., Murray, T. J., Seland, T. P., Duquette, P., Grey, T., Nelson, R., Nicolle, M., and Brunet, D. "A Population-Based Study of Multiple Sclerosis in Twins." *New England Journal of Medicine,* 1986, *315,* 1638-1642.

Federal Register. *Developmental Disabilities Act of 1984.* Report 981074, Section 102 (11F), 1984.

Franklin, G. M., Nelson, L. M., Heaton, R. K., Burks, J. S., and Thompson, D. S. "Stress and Its Relationship to Acute Exacerbations in Multiple Sclerosis." *Journal of Neurologic Rehabilitation,* 1988, *2,* 7-11.

Genevie, L., Kallos, J. E., and Struening, E. L. "Job Retention Among People with Multiple Sclerosis." *Journal of Neurologic Rehabilitation,* 1987, *1,* 131-135.

Grant, I., Brown, G. W., Harris, T., McDonald, W. I., Patterson, T., and Trimble, M. R. "Severely Threatening Events and Marked Life Difficulties Preceding Onset or Exacerbations of Multiple Sclerosis." *Journal of Neurology, Neurosurgery, and Psychiatry,* 1989, *52,* 8-13.

Hammond, S. R., English, D., de Wytt, C., Maxwell, I. C., Millingen, K. S., Stewart-Wynne, E. G., McLeod, J. G., and McCall, M. G. "The Clinical Profile of MS in Australia: A Comparison Between Medium- and High-Frequency Prevalence Zones." *Neurology,* 1988, *38,* 980-986.

Kallos, J. E., Genevie, L., Struening, E. L., and Andrews, H. F. "The Role of

Advocacy Groups in Vocational Rehabilitation Service Delivery to the Severely Disabled: A Comparison Between Multiple Sclerosis and Other Disorders." *Journal of Neurologic Rehabilitation,* 1988, *2,* 13–20.

Kornblith, A. B., LaRocca, N. G., and Baum, H. M. "Employment in Individuals with Multiple Sclerosis." *International Journal of Rehabilitation Research,* 1986, *9,* 155–165.

Kraft, G. H., Freal, J. E., Coryell, J. K., Hanan, B. S., and Chitnis, N. "Multiple Sclerosis: Early Prognostic Guidelines." *Archives of Physical Medicine and Rehabilitation,* 1981, *62,* 54–58.

LaRocca, N. G. "Psychosocial Factors in Multiple Sclerosis and the Role of Stress." In L. C. Scheinberg and C. S. Raine (eds.), *Multiple Sclerosis: Experimental and Clinical Aspects. Annals of the New York Academy of Sciences.* New York: New York Academy of Sciences, 1984.

LaRocca, N. G., Kalb, R., Scheinberg, L. C., and Kendall, P. "Factors Associated with Unemployment of Patients with Multiple Sclerosis." *Journal of Chronic Diseases,* 1985, *38,* 203–210.

National Association of Rehabilitation Facilities. "PWI Evaluation Positive." *NARF Rehabilitation Review,* vol. 3, 1986.

National Multiple Sclerosis Society, Rehabilitation Services Administration, and The Council of State Administrators of Vocational Rehabilitation. "Joint Statement of Principles." Unpublished report, 1978.

National Multiple Sclerosis Society, Rehabilitation Services Administration, National Institute of Handicapped Research, and The Council of State Administrators of Vocational Rehabilitation. "Cooperative Agreement." Unpublished report, 1983.

Paty, D. W., and Poser, C. M. "Clinical Symptoms and Signs of Multiple Sclerosis." In C. M. Poser, D. W. Paty, L. C. Scheinberg, W. I. McDonald, and G. C. Ebers (eds.), *The Diagnosis of Multiple Sclerosis.* New York: Thieme-Stratton, 1984.

Pavlou, M. M. *Variety and Possibility in Multiple Sclerosis.* Chicago: Bio Service Corp., 1979.

Rabkin, J. G. "Stress and Psychiatric Disorders." In L. Goldberger and S. Breznitz (eds.), *Handbook of Stress: Theoretical and Clinical Aspects.* New York: Free Press, 1982.

Rao, S. M. "Neuropsychology of Multiple Sclerosis: A Critical Review." *Journal of Clinical and Experimental Neuropsychology,* 1986, *8,* 503–542.

Rao, S. M. "Impact of Cognitive Dysfunction on Employment and Social Functioning in MS Patients." Paper presented at the annual meeting of the American Academy of Neurology, April 1989.

Sadovnick, A. D., and Baird, P. A. "The Familial Nature of Multiple Sclerosis: Age-Corrected Empiric Recurrence Risks for Children and Siblings of Patients." *Neurology,* 1988, *38,* 990–991.

Scheinberg, L. C. *Model Program for the Comprehensive Vocational Rehabilitation of Multiple Sclerosis Patients.* Rehabilitation Services Administration Grant 30-P-65161A/2-02, 1978.

Scheinberg, L. C. *Comprehensive Continuing Care and Rehabilitative Program for Multiple Sclerosis Patients.* National Institute for Handicapped Research Grant G008006808, 1980.

Scheinberg, L. C., Holland, N. J., LaRocca, N. G., Laitin, P., Bennett, A., and Hall, H. L. "Multiple Sclerosis: Earning a Living." *New York State Journal of Medicine,* 1980, *80,* 1395–1400.

Social Security Administration. *A Summary Guide to Social Security and Supple-*

mental Security Income Work Incentives for the Disabled and Blind. Baltimore, Md.: Social Security Administration Office of Disability, 1988.

Stevens, J. R. "Schizophrenia and Multiple Sclerosis." *Schizophrenia Bulletin,* 1988, *14,* 231-241.

Nicholas G. LaRocca, Ph.D., is associate professor of neurology (psychology) at the Albert Einstein College of Medicine. He is director of research within the Medical Rehabilitation Research and Training Center for Multiple Sclerosis and deputy director for administration of the Rehabilitation Research and Training Center for Psychiatrically Disabled Individuals.

Harry L. Hall has served as an associate commissioner of the Rehabilitation Services Administration and Washington Representative of the National MS Society. He is currently president of The Development Team, Inc., a not-for-profit corporation involved in delivering employment services to persons with chronic disabilities, particularly MS.

New sources and methods are necessary to finance housing for people with long-term mental illness. This chapter describes an innovative program to increase the amount of capital available for such housing.

New Funding Strategy for Housing for People with Mental Disabilities

Leonard S. Rubenstein, Linda B. James

Permanent and affordable housing remains one of the most basic unmet needs of persons with a mental illness. Shorter hospital stays, successful community-based treatment, and respect for the liberty of the individual cannot be achieved without a stable and supportive community living environment. Yet many of the estimated 1.7 to 2.4 million Americans considered to be suffering from "long-term mental illnesses" based on psychiatric diagnosis, severity of disability, and duration of disorder are inadequately or inappropriately housed or homeless (Goldman, Gattozzi, and Taube, 1981).

The decline in the stock of low-income housing is well documented and especially devastating for mentally ill people. The number of single-room occupancy hotels, a traditional source of housing for deinstitutionalized mental patients, was reduced by 50 percent from 1970 to 1980. According to a recent study, the shortage of affordable housing has increased by over 2.15 million units, or 120 percent, since 1980, and only a very small number of these units are replaced each year (National Low-Income Housing Coalition, 1986; Randolph, Laux, and Carling, 1987). During this same period, public-sector support for housing subsidies sharply declined. As a result, there is rigorous competition for available housing resources, and people with a record of mental illness face historic discrimination in the selection process. At the same time, dramatically increasing housing costs have rendered generation of new housing for low-income people extremely difficult, so that private developers have left the low-income housing arena. People with special needs stand even farther outside this shrinking resource pool.

Developers of low-income housing, beset by problems in financing and managing their projects, frequently shy away from a population with a reputation for being difficult. They know little of the needs or desires of the people who are expected to live in the units or how to provide appropriate and individualized services for them. Community mental health agencies, though adept at providing the services, usually lack experience in housing development. After a decade in which the federal housing budget was cut by 70 percent, money for development is hard to find. Those funds that are available often come with regulations that defeat objectives such as normalization and community integration.

To overcome these obstacles, those who wish to develop housing must find new sources of capital, use those sources to leverage additional subsidies, utilize the expertise of nonprofit agencies that are experienced in developing low-income housing, and create ways to provide individualized services while encouraging autonomy for people with mental disabilities. This chapter describes one such effort: the use of back-benefit awards under the Social Security Disability Insurance (SSDI) and the Supplemental Security Income (SSI) disability programs for permanent housing. Although the most unique aspect of this project concerns a new source of financing—capital contributions by individuals who will live in the units—the housing program may also help illuminate how to plan for the integration of housing and services for people with major mental illness.

Using Back-Benefit Awards to Finance Housing

Litigation. The project's origins had nothing to do with housing. In the late 1970s and early 1980s, the Social Security Administration ushered in new but undisclosed rules for assessing disability claims of people with psychiatric impairments. Under the new rules, the evaluation of a claimant's actual ability to work as required by law was replaced by formulas that had no basis in medicine, rehabilitation research, or law (Rubenstein, Gattozzi, and Goldman, 1988; Rubenstein, 1985). The rules were put into effect at the same time as the Social Security Administration embarked on congressionally mandated reviews of the eligibility of thousands of disability beneficiaries—reviews the newly installed Reagan Administration accelerated in anticipation of huge savings (Goldman and Gattozzi, 1988). The results were catastrophic: Between mid-1981 and mid-1983 more than 100,000 mentally ill people were denied or terminated from benefits.

Lawsuits challenged these and other unlawful policies employed by the Social Security Administration (SSA). One of these suits, *City of New York* v. *Heckler,* was filed in early 1983 on behalf of all disability claimants with severe psychiatric impairments in New York State. A year later, the court ruled in the plaintiffs' favor and ordered the reopening of all New York State claims involving disability as a result of severe psychotic or nonpsychotic mental disorders between early 1980 and mid-1983 (*City of New York* v. *Heckler,* 1984).

No cases were reopened, however, while the government appealed the decision. This meant that, except for people who had reapplied and been found eligible, the amount of claimants' potential back-benefit awards kept increasing. The government's appeal was not resolved until June of 1986 (*Bowen* v. *City of New York,* 1986), and it took another year to identify the 14,700 individual victims in New York State, find accurate addresses, and agree on procedures for reopening the cases. Another two years were consumed in locating class members, shepherding them through the reopening procedures, monitoring the adjudication of the cases, and resolving the myriad glitches that occurred along the way.

The delays brought the average back-benefit award to more than $14,000. Awards of double that amount were common. But for recipients of SSI, the awards came with a catch: As a means-tested welfare program, SSI allowed a recipient to possess only $1800 in nonexempt resources. The law allowed an exception for recipients of back-benefit awards, but only a small one: They were permitted six months to spend the award down to $1800. If, after that time, an unmarried recipient possessed resources in excess of the $1800 maximum allowed, he or she would be terminated from current benefits.

One solution to this paradox was to extend the time in which to dispose of the resources. Congress, however, agreed to a temporary extension of only nine months. Another alternative was to figure a way to convert the funds to a nonexempt resource. Under the SSI rules, one's own home is the most significant allowable resource. Thus a strategy evolved: to help class members invest their back-benefit awards in a housing arrangement. With the support of the Robert Wood Johnson Foundation and the cooperation of the Social Security Administration, the Mental Health Law Project, a nonprofit national public-interest organization, undertook this effort.

Implementation of the Lawsuit. In 1987, the Mental Health Law Project initiated a social security entitlement and housing program in New York State (MHLP/NY) to implement the *City of New York* decision and enable interested claimants to use their back benefits for housing. MHLP/NY has conducted concurrent efforts to (1) identify class members and assist them with their claims through an outreach program designed to enlist the services of public agencies throughout the state and (2) develop a plan for class members to use their back benefits to meet their long-term housing needs. The results to date demonstrate that vigorous outreach, support, and legal assistance significantly increase the number of claimants who actually claim and receive retroactive benefits. The review rate of *City of New York* claims to date far exceeds the rate reported by the Social Security Administration for most other disability cases. SSA reports a standard award rate of 36 percent; from a low of 37 percent in January 1988, *City of New York* claims in April 1989 resulted in awards at a rate of 77 percent.

During the outreach program, MHLP/NY learned that many class members are either homeless or housed in substandard conditions and that their single most important priority is safe, affordable, and permanent housing. To respond to the critical need for affordable housing, MHLP/NY developed a low-income supportive housing model that utilizes the investment of the back-benefit awards. The plan proposes three components: (1) a housing development fund, an independent nonprofit corporation serving as a repository for funds from class members and other investors and as a source of capital financing for development projects, (2) a housing development corporation, an independent corporation to serve as a developer and/or joint-venturer for housing projects statewide, and (3) a consumer services agency to identify and link consumers' housing needs to housing and support services.

The key element in this innovative housing program is a national demonstration agreement negotiated with the Social Security Administration. The terms of the agreement provide that retroactive SSDI and SSI benefits paid to class members may be voluntarily contributed to a housing development fund and pooled with funds from state and local governments and private investors in order to build, renovate, and lease housing throughout New York State. The fund is permitted to receive class members' awards and apply them to planned housing projects without invoking the SSA spend-down rules. Rather, under the terms of the demonstration project, SSA will suspend certain SSI income and resources counting rules while these funds are held by the development fund for use in providing affordable housing.

As stated in the Federal Register notice (Vol. 54, No. 134, July 14, 1989), the objectives of SSA participation in this demonstration project are twofold. First, it will assist certain mentally disabled SSI recipients in the State of New York who were class members in *Bowen* v. *City of New York* in meeting their shelter needs, thereby fulfilling one of the purposes of the SSI program. Second, it will permit class members who are homeless or are living in marginal housing to use their retroactive benefits to obtain permanent housing and supportive services without affecting their SSI eligibility or payment amount, thereby enabling them to function as autonomously and productively as possible. Class members have the option to withdraw their money from the fund up to the end of the demonstration project in 1992. After this time, withdrawal of funds by class members is contingent on the particular arrangement made.

Housing Development Fund. There is a need for creative financing in the development of supportive housing for mentally ill people, including opportunities that allow the timely purchase of property for future development, housing construction loans from a single source, and permanent loan terms that allow the developer or owner to offer affordable rents while permitting the fund a reasonable rate of return. In addition to facing the same problems confronting the private sector, nonprofit developers face restrictive cycles in government funding and loan terms from conventional leaders that affect the affordability of rents.

The Mental Health Law Project has established a nonprofit development fund, Access Housing Development Fund, as the repository for class-member back benefits. The purpose of the fund is to promote low-income supportive housing development through financial support, in the form of grants, loans, and guaranties; and technical assistance, in leveraging additional financing from either public or private sources. The fund will pool the investments by *City of New York* class members, in accordance with the national demonstration agreement authorized by the Social Security Administration, and will generate additional capital to finance the production of low-income supportive housing. In addition to the class-member investments, the fund's capital will be raised from financial institutions, corporations, foundations, government agencies, and private investors, such as families with mentally ill members.

The resources held by the fund will provide new sources of capital to stimulate the production of low-income supportive housing. The fund will reduce the need to deal with a multiplicity of funding cycles in financing low-income projects. The fund will make loans from the capital pool to qualifying organizations, coordinate diverse financing sources for all developers who meet the loan criteria, and raise additional funds from those governmental and private sources that require or prefer nonprofit sponsorship and/or central administration for "special needs" housing development projects.

The fund will participate in the financing of tenant-occupied, owner-occupied, and mixed-use residential or commercial projects. The fund will use financial strategies to capitalize projects such as pooling equity investments or leveraging additional financing in the production of appropriate housing properties, providing below-market interest rate loans to special-needs housing developers for pre-development, construction, bridge and permanent financing. It will also act as a financial and technical assistance intermediary to package public resources with private-sector equity funds in the production of low-income supportive housing.

Clients of the fund will be nonprofit organizations and private developers who are committed to respond to the housing needs of mentally ill people in New York State. The fund will not own, develop, or manage land or residential properties. Maintenance of rental affordability will be a primary requirement for any project in which the fund makes a financial investment. The fund will work closely with each developer to structure and negotiate the terms of the project's financing.

Housing Development Corporation. Successful expansion of low-income supportive housing stock will require financing arrangements as well as the capacity to manage the real estate development process. Nonprofit organizations interested in and willing to own and manage special-needs housing may not want to develop the property. The housing development corporation is being established to assist the projects supported by the development fund during the production process. In this capacity it will identify development opportunities for special-needs housing, create housing development partnerships or co-ventures for the production of supportive housing, and initiate the production of units that integrate mental health and support services into the design of the housing program.

As a developer of low-income supportive housing units for mentally ill people, the housing development corporation will identify potential housing stock and sites, develop a housing and financing plan for the site selected, select and direct architectural and other technical project consultants, supervise the construction phases of a project, prepare buildings for occupancy, and coordinate the social services program planning with the developer and the community and coordinate the tenant selection process and management plans.

Housing arrangements to be considered include single-room occupancies (SROs), apartments, and private and multifamily homes, depending on the characteristics of the particular community, the availability of existing stock, the needs and financial resources of community nonprofit organizations, and other factors.

Supportive Housing Services. For many people who are mentally ill, long-term stable living situations are feasible only if appropriate support services are provided to meet their needs. At the outset of the development process, planning must begin to link the residential needs of the mentally ill consumer with individually appropriate social services. Working in conjunction with a consumer services unit, the fund and the development corporation will use the consumer services expertise of the Mental Health Law Project and the MHLP/NY outreach program to include appropriate social services program elements in each of the funds' projects.

Services are intended for individuals who have a history of mental illness and resulting functional disabilities. Each program will be tailored to the ambiance of the residence and to the needs and requests of the tenants. A range of services will be offered including outreach, screening, case management, legal referrals, entitlement reviews, individual and group therapy, medication monitoring, socialization, and recreational activities. Each program will address the total rehabilitation needs of residents based on functional assessments and individual choice and will encourage participation in a variety of on-site and off-site activities. The programs will help maintain and develop those life skills necessary to enable residents to function at the highest possible level in their environment as well as to establish and maintain community service linkages.

Evaluation, Limitations, and Implications

The project we have described depended upon unique circumstances: the availability of substantial back-benefit awards to a large group of people known to the developer. But although nonduplicable in the narrow sense, the project offers some significant lessons about housing development for people with mental disabilities.

Strategy. A pooled investment fund to generate new sources of low-cost financing for community development corporations and other low-income housing developers is not new. Direct financial support through loans, grants, and equity investment by The Enterprise Foundation and Local Initiatives Support Corporation (LISC) have underwritten low-income housing development and community renewal throughout the country. However, neither organization has performed these activities for special-needs housing development. The proposed fund is unique in the low-income housing development marketplace because it (1) is dedicated to a special-needs population, (2) has nationwide replicability because it is part of a Social Security Administration demonstration project, (3) provides the opportunity for interested recipients of Social Security back benefits to invest their own equity in permanent housing, and (4) creates a link with a consumer service agency as a resource to match consumer needs with supportive services.

New York State housing production plans over the next five years include the rehabilitation of over 300 city-owned units, 100 suburban units financed through the development fund, and 50 to 100 units in upstate New York financed through local corporate partnerships. In each area, the housing fund has identified and developed new sources of financing to help provide the housing. The common denominator in each has been the class-member investment of Social Security back benefits.

Changes Needed in the SSI Program. Like other means-tested welfare programs, SSI contains financial eligibility criteria so complex as to mimic the Internal Revenue Code. It took more than a year of negotiation before SSA finally approved the use of funds for the purposes we have described, and only then by a demonstration project that relieved SSA of the obligation of determining whether the project fit within existing rules.

At least two SSI eligibility rules prevent people from obtaining decent housing. First, and most important, except for income or resource subsidies a recipient obtains to promote ownership of a home, SSI counts any nonpublic subsidy, including a person's own resources, used to help pay for one's housing as income or a resource, depending on the circumstances of receipt. This policy means that rent-supplement payments made by family, churches, charitable institutions, or any other nongovernmental entity will, in most cases, reduce the SSI grant almost dollar for dollar. Ownership or equity interests in housing no doubt should be encouraged, but no penalty ought to be applied for reasonable and limited private assistance enabling a person to obtain housing. Unless SSI benefit levels are raised sufficiently to permit the grant to cover actual rental costs, SSI rules ought affirmatively to allow reasonable rental subsidies by others.

Second, the brief time allowed people to "spend down" back-benefit awards discourages people from being able to use the funds for a housing investment. The "use it or lose it" rules have other defects, too, such as encouraging financial profligacy. But it is particularly tragic that recipients are not given enough time to turn a windfall into an investment. The most logical rule would be to exclude back-benefit awards from resources altogether, since the money is not a personal resource in the true sense but rather the lump-sum repayment of a prior debt incurred over time owed by the government to the recipient.

Implications of the Project. Can the lessons of this project be utilized elsewhere? We believe they can.

The central feature of the project was the ability to aggregate relatively small contributions, use the aggregated funds to leverage additional subsidies, and develop housing. The source of the funds does not matter. They may come from future residents' back-benefit awards, bequests, or other sources. They may come from an even more likely source: the members of recipients' own families. Or they may come from small charitable contributions. What does matter is that a vehicle exists to collect the funds and use the capital to stimulate housing development. We were, in fact, surprised at the leveraging effect of this source of capital—that is, how much easier it was to gain access to other sources of development money by having the relatively small contributions available or likely to be made available.

Use of the Social Security back benefit as an effective resource in the competitive housing development marketplace provides a new and creative source of capital to stimulate the production of low-income supportive housing. Investment in a development fund created through a Social Security national demonstration agreement allows the individual investor to become an equity holder in his or her living arrangement. The back benefit becomes an investment in the permanence of a supportive setting in a community in which the mentally ill person becomes a participating member with a meaningful social role. The opportunity for each individual to make a contribution to his or her community becomes a reality.

References

Bowen v. *City of New York,* 476 U.S. 467 (1986).

City of New York v. *Heckler,* 578 F. Supp. 1109 (E.D.N.Y. 1984), *aff'd* 742 F.2d 729 (2d Cir. 1985), *aff'd sub nom. Bowen* v. *City of New York,* 476 U.S. 467 (1986).

Goldman, H. H., and Gattozzi, A. "Murder in the Cathedral Revisited: President Reagan and the Mentally Disabled." *Hospital and Community Psychiatry,* 1988, *39,* 505–509.

Goldman, H. H., Gattozzi, A. A., and Taube, C. "Defining and Counting the Chronically Mentally Ill." *Hospital and Community Psychiatry,* 1981, *32,* 21–27.

National Low-Income Housing Coalition. *Rental Crisis Deepens for Low-Income Renters.* Washington, D.C.: National Low Income Housing Coalition, 1986.

Randolph, F. L., Laux, B., and Carling, P. J. *In Search of Housing.* Boston: Center for Psychiatric Rehabilitation, Boston University, and Center for Community Change Through Housing and Support, University of Vermont, 1987.

Rubenstein, L. S. "Science, Law, and Psychiatric Disability." *Psychosocial Rehabilitation Journal,* 1985, *9,* 7–19.

Rubenstein, L. S. Gattozzi, A. A., and Goldman, H. H. "Protecting the Entitlements of the Mentally Disabled: The SSDI/SSI Legal Battles of the 1980s." *International Journal of Law and Psychiatry,* 1988, *11,* 269–278.

Leonard S. Rubenstein is legal director of the Mental Health Law Project and was one of the counsel for the class in Bowen *v.* City of New York.

Linda B. James is the director of the Access Housing Development Fund referred to in this chapter and is director of Housing Development in the Mental Health Law Project's New York office.

With annual national health spending already at $400 billion and alarming numbers of chronically mentally ill individuals critically needing multiple services, how does one philanthropic foundation find a way to help?

The Robert Wood Johnson Foundation Mental Health Services Development Program

Leonard I. Stein

During the past thirty years there have been dramatic changes in the way mentally ill people are treated. Largely because of deinstitutionalization, the resident population of public mental hospitals in the United States has been reduced by more than 70 percent. As a result, thousands of people with chronic mental illness, who in years past would have been long-term residents of public mental institutions, now live in community settings. Much has been learned about the kinds of programs needed to help persons with chronic mental illness make a stable and satisfactory adjustment to living in the community. However, programs have developed slowly, and thus in most parts of the nation, patients are receiving inadequate care.

In response to this problem, The Robert Wood Johnson Foundation created the Mental Health Services Development Program. Initiated in 1987, the project supports state and local initiatives designed to improve access to a broad range of health care and community services for the chronically mentally ill. A $10 million competitive program was structured in three rounds of funding, and is providing grants of up to $600,000 each for eighteen projects.

This chapter reviews the experience to date of the Mental Health Services Development Program, giving some background information

---

The views expressed in this article are those of the author. No endorsement by The Robert Wood Johnson Foundation is intended or should be inferred.

on The Robert Wood Johnson Foundation's creation of this program. It also outlines the grant procedures and priority considerations of the program, as well as briefly describes the program's eighteen funded projects.

The Robert Wood Johnson Foundation

The Robert Wood Johnson Foundation is now the largest health foundation in the country and has made grants totaling over $750 million. The following statistics help put this into perspective. In the United States, there are some 23,000 foundations having total resources of $50 billion and making grants totaling nearly $4 billion per year (Nielsen, 1985). The United States is unique in the utilization of private grant-making foundations. In the area of health, private foundations invest over $700 million a year. Although this may seem like a large amount of money, it is minuscule in comparison to the annual national expenditure of $387 billion a year, of which $112 billion comes from federal health outlays (Levit, Lazenby, Waldo, and Davidoff, 1985). Thus, private foundations account for less than one-half of 1 percent of the total health expenditures.

At the present time, The Robert Wood Johnson Foundation is making grants totaling approximately $100 million per year (Robert Wood Johnson Foundation annual report, 1987) for health and health-related projects. However, compared to the nearly $400 billion being expended annually for health care in this country, $100 million had to be carefully targeted in order to make a significant impact on the health scene. Thus, when it came to making decisions about where it would spend its money, the Foundation made a careful analysis of expenditures by other foundations and the federal government in the health care area. Essentially, they found that adding the Foundation's funds to what was being spent for biomedical research would only increase the biomedical research budget by 1 percent. However, if Foundation funds were added to the budget being spent by the federal government in health care delivery research, it would increase that budget by 53 percent. Thus, the major thrust would be in the area of health care delivery.

The three specific target issues defined for health care delivery efforts to be supported by the Foundation were

1. Improving access to personal health care for the most underserved population groups
2. Helping to make health care arrangements more effective and more affordable
3. Enhancing individuals' capacities to function effectively in everyday life.

Congruent with these three areas, the Foundation has supported a variety of service, training, and research programs. The mental health area, however, is a newcomer to The Robert Wood Johnson Foundation. Their first initiative in this area was the Program for the Chronically Mentally Ill. This effort was directed toward cities that have a population of over 250,000. A national competition was held, and nine cities were selected for funding. The thrust of this initiative was primarily toward system change to bring about better care for the chronically mentally ill (Aiken, Somers, and Shore, 1986).

Their second initiative, the Mental Health Services Development Program, was designed to support both comprehensive and more targeted efforts to improve access to appropriate services for chronically mentally ill people. Specifically, the program supports development and implementation of demonstration projects concerned with financing and service-delivery arrangements at the state and local levels.

Process Used to Select Grantees

Approximately 10,000 requests for proposals were distributed to virtually every eligible entity that had an interest in the chronically mentally ill. The application process was quite straightforward and much simpler than proposals required by most federal agencies. The proposal was limited to twenty double-spaced pages, exclusive of budget and résumés of project personnel. The proposal needed to include the following:

1. A discussion of the problem the project would address in improving access to care for chronically mentally ill individuals
2. A detailed description of the proposed project
3. A discussion of how the project would assist in solving the identified problem
4. Evidence that the proposed project had the active support and endorsement of relevant groups
5. Discussion of any barriers specific to the project that must be overcome before implementation
6. Estimated overall effect of the project, including the number of chronically mentally ill people to be served, the geographic area to be involved, and the anticipated outcomes to be achieved
7. A time frame for project development and implementation
8. Plans for continuation of the project following the grant period
9. The qualifications and expertise of those responsible for planning and implementing the project
10. A budget, including a budget narrative.

The procedure was structured to provide three rounds of funding. The first deadline for receipt of applications was February 1, 1987; the second, June 1, 1987; and the third, December 1, 1987. Over the three periods, 271 proposals were received.

The standard operating procedure for the Robert Wood Johnson Foundation's national program initiatives is to have a review panel made up of experts in the area who represent the professions that may be involved in the projects and who come from various parts of the country. Professions represented on the review panel for the Mental Health Services Development Program were: psychiatry, social work, psychology, nursing, and sociology. Expertise among those professions included clinical intervention, research methodology, administration at the state level, administration at the agency level, housing, and systems issues. Advisory to the review panel were representatives from the Foundation, a representative from the National Institute of Mental Health (NIMH), and a representative from the Program for the Chronically Mentally Ill.

For each round, the proposals were first reviewed by the program director of the Mental Health Services Development Program and by the two Foundation officers involved in the program. They selected approximately 25 percent of each round's incoming proposals to be forwarded to the review panel for further consideration. Thus, for each round, approximately twenty-five proposals were sent to each review-panel member for consideration. Each panel member was to score each proposal on a scale from one to five, based on the following considerations:

1. The numbers of chronically mentally ill persons who could ultimately be affected by the project
2. The feasibility of the proposal's being operationalized
3. The probability of its continuing once the grant funding ceased
4. The degree of innovation of the program
5. The potential replicability of the project in other parts of the country.

After scoring each proposal, the panel members forwarded their scores to the national program office. Approximately one-fourth of the proposals' authors were selected to come to a meeting of the review panel for a face-to-face discussion.

After each round, the review panel met, along with its before-mentioned advisers, and discussed all proposals reviewed by the panel in that round. Following discussion, the representatives selected to defend their proposals were interviewed separately. After the interviews, the panel then voted on which proposals they would recommend to the Foundation's Board of Trustees for funding. From the total of 271 proposals, eighteen were funded. The following sections provide descriptions of the eighteen projects.

Systems Change Projects

"Fulfilling the Vision: Completion of the Community-Based System in Vermont" (The Regionalization Project). State of Vermont Department of Mental Health, Waterbury, Vermont. The Regionalization Project is in the final phase of a twenty-five year shift from institutional to community-based mental health care in Vermont. Since the passage of the Community Mental Health Services Act in 1963, ten Community Mental Health Centers (CMHCs) have offered local alternatives to institutionalization. During the same years, the state's centralized public institution, Vermont State Hospital (VSH) has served a declining average daily population, from over 1,200 twenty-five years ago to approximately 190 at the beginning of the present project.

This project, then, is directed toward demonstrating that an entire state can virtually terminate its use of the state hospital by completing the development of a statewide system of integrated community services. Vermont is progressing well in its goal of reducing the population of Vermont State Hospital to eighty nursing home, forensic, and long-term patients while developing, improving, and restructuring services designed to meet the needs of most individuals with prolonged, severe mental illness, emphasizing the provision of community-based crisis services as well as housing, vocational, and related supports.

The Assertive Community Treatment Service (ACTS), State of Connecticut Department of Mental Health, Hartford, Connecticut. The ACTS project is a system-wide effort to develop a model that will coordinate services for the chronically mentally ill throughout the state's five service-delivery regions (made up of 158 different agencies contracted by the State Department of Mental Health) in such a way that services are made available at a single point of responsibility. Because ACTS focuses on those "at risk" persons with prolonged mental illness who use a high percentage of services and require frequent hospitalizations, it features intensive and responsive service provided by an interdisciplinary team familiar with the clients, their needs, and their difficulties in managing the current service system. The team coordinates a wide range of community services, provides twenty-four-hour crisis intervention and case management, and develops strong support systems both with the family and throughout the community in an effort to avoid unnecessary, restrictive, and expensive hospitalization.

Drawing on the experiences of similar models designed and implemented in other parts of the country, and combining this with their knowledge of local needs and resources and their capacity for analysis and evaluation, the Department of Mental Health (DMH) is working to create a model program that will demonstrate how a cohesive, managed service system can be implemented statewide.

System Integration and Specialized Services for People with Chronic Mental Illness and Substance Abuse Problems. State of New Hampshire, Division of Mental Health & Development Services, Concord, New Hampshire. The majority of mental health inpatient and outpatient programs designed to treat seriously mentally ill individuals have not paid attention to providing treatment that will interrupt the cycle of mental illness and substance abuse. Historically, these persons have presented numerous diagnostic and treatment approach challenges. Although a mentally ill person may be stabilized relatively quickly, that gain can quickly be lost because of the person's continued reliance on alcohol and other drugs. Thus, New Hampshire's Division of Mental Health and Developmental Services, through the community mental health centers located throughout the state, is developing an integrated approach to treating individuals with these dual disabilities. Major emphases are placed on close collaboration and coordination between service providers, assurances of continuity of care, and cross-training for mental health and substance abuse professionals. The project centers provision of services to this population on the development of two major initiatives: (1) specialized treatment teams in all ten regions of New Hampshire, and (2) two short-term residential facilities serving the entire state.

Housing, Outreach and Employment Project (HOEP). Rhode Island Department of Mental Health, Retardation and Hospitals, Division of Mental Health & Community Support Services, Cranston, Rhode Island. The Housing, Outreach and Employment Project (HOEP) is a threefold demonstration project that combines and improves services for psychiatrically disabled adults from the ages of eighteen to forty. The project is implementing supportive programs to address each major domain of clients' lives: where and how they live, work, and receive treatment. Cross-catchment-area, mobile community treatment teams provide aggressive outreach and treatment in residences, hospitals, and jails to these psychiatrically disabled young adults with mental illness, substance abuse, or legal problems. Through HOEP and other residential initiatives, an array of residential services is being planned and implemented across the state for these clients. Clients can choose from an expanded spectrum of supported employment options that range from food service and other industries to new vocational agencies serving the project area.

The initial project site, located in the Northeastern quadrant of Rhode Island, encompasses two catchment areas, each of which is served by separate community mental health centers. One mobile treatment team has been developed to serve this area, involving about sixty clients in its first year of operation. This interagency collaborative effort builds upon the strengths of Rhode Island's mental health system and makes possible a much wider array of service. HOEP's innovative program will serve as a model for further systems change statewide and nationally.

Homeless Projects

LAMP Village, Los Angeles, California. LAMP has offered drop-in, community-based services to the homeless, chronically mentally ill on the Los Angeles Skid Row since June 1985. This safe, accessible program attracts hardcore and noncompliant mentally ill men who have been caught up in an endless cycle of living on the streets, going to jail, or going into twenty-four- to seventy-two-hour psychiatric holds and returning to the street with little or no follow-up.

LAMP's Village project consists of two components: a transitioning residence for forty-eight homeless, chronically mentally ill men and women, and cottage industries that will provide entry-level and skilled employment, as well as job training, for these men and women, most of whom have never had the opportunity to work because of their mental illness. The aims of the project include: goal-oriented residential treatment for forty-eight men and women lasting several weeks to several months; up to ten beds reserved for residents who are dual diagnosed; case management, medication, and money management; in-house health and mental health screenings; coordination of psychiatric treatment provided by the county's Skid Row Mental Health Clinic located a half block away from the Village; and advocacy assistance in obtaining and maintaining economic benefits, health treatment, and permanent housing.

Arraignment Court Diversion Program, Los Angeles County Department of Mental Health, Forensic Mental Health Services Bureau, Los Angeles, California. A growing number of chronically mentally ill people are being inappropriately housed in jail, owing mainly to dwindling public resources and inadequate community-based mental health treatment systems. These clients both contribute to and suffer enormously from the general problem of jail and court system overcrowding.

This project aims to address these problems within Los Angeles County by hiring staff who identify mentally ill misdemeanor offenders at the point of jail system entry (Arraignment Court), provide careful psychiatric assessment and crisis intervention, and, when possible, divert the mentally ill from the legal system to appropriate mental health and community support services. The program includes intense, daily interaction of mental health staff with court and legal staff to assure timely and appropriate placements of the mentally ill. The program also provides an extensive follow-up case management program to assure continuity of care to mentally ill persons who are diverted from the jail system to the mental health system.

Clinical Case Management/Mobile Outreach Unit, University of Medicine and Dentistry of New Jersey, Community Mental Health Center at Piscataway, New Brunswick, New Jersey. This project is designed to work with an emerging group of seriously mentally ill adults who are not being adequately served by existing emergency treatment, outpatient and day-treatment services in the community. These clients require innovative and flexible clinical case management and assertive and mobile outreach services in order to reduce inappropriate inpatient treatment and to provide quality mental health services where none existed previously. Staff of this project regularly visit the county shelters, rooming houses, apartments, street locations, and homes to provide evaluation, referral, and treatment services. Clients who meet the criteria for the clinical case management services from within the service area are being referred to this project. Clinical case management services are provided indefinitely based upon need rather than performance of the client. Mobile outreach is available to project clients on an as-needed basis.

Project Interlink, Travelers & Immigrants Aid, Health Care for the Homeless, Chicago, Illinois. Project Interlink is a collaboration between the Health Care for the Homeless Connections Program of Travelers and Immigrants Aid, which provides outreach to shelters, drop-in centers, the streets, and inpatient psychiatric facilities, and Thresholds Bridge for the Homeless, which provides assertive long-term case management. The target population is the homeless mentally ill who are difficult to engage, resistant to services, and initially unable or unwilling to maintain housing and mental health linkages. Clients are pervasively impaired in their ability to manage the most basic daily living tasks, and show little or no improvement once they are resettled. Specific criteria for referral to Project Interlink are the following:

1. Difficult engagement process wherein the clients' resistance and elusiveness indicate a severe impairment in their ability to become involved in a case-management regimen.
2. History and/or current demonstration of severe mental illness, chronic or episodic homelessness, and inability to make use of most basic resources, including funding, food, clothing, and health care. Resettlement does not improve functioning or psychiatric symptoms.
3. Symptomatology is severe and pervasive enough that money management, adherence to minimal housing regulations, and linkage with mental health services is not likely without ongoing, long-term case management.

Once a client is assessed by Connections staff to be appropriate for Project Interlink, Bridge team members begin working with him or her in all case management activities.

Housing Projects

Program to Substantially Expand Therapeutic Housing Arrangements, Mental Health Law Project, Washington, D.C. This project was designed in response to the 1986 decision by the U.S. Supreme Court in *Bowen* v. *City of New York,* which found that at least 14,000 mentally ill people in New York State were entitled to claim back benefits because they had been improperly deprived of Social Security Disability Insurance (SSDI) or Supplemental Security Income (SSI) between April 1, 1980, and May 14, 1983.

Because of the acute shortage of affordable, decent housing available to low-income mentally disabled people, this project was developed to use the back Social Security benefits awarded as a result of the class action *City of New York* decision to develop housing opportunities for persons covered by this court action. The project was designed to pursue two separate but related efforts: (1) outreach activities to all individuals potentially affected by the *City of New York* decision; and (2) housing development through investment by class members of their back-benefit payments in a mutual housing association.

By the end of the two-year grant period, this project expects to have designed a model for investment of back Social Security benefits or other lump-sum payments received by seriously mentally ill individuals that can substantially expand therapeutic housing for low-income people who are mentally ill. A full report of the model will be distributed to providers and advocates serving mentally ill people throughout the nation.

Clustered Apartment Project, County of Santa Clara Mental Health Bureau, Community Support Subsystem, San Jose, California. The Clustered Apartment Project takes as its primary task the development and maintenance of permanent housing and a reliable social support system for people in Santa Clara County who are assessed as seriously mentally ill. It is intended to serve people now found at all levels of the residential care continuum. This includes people in Transitional Residential programs, Supported Independent Living programs, and Board and Care homes, as well as those who are in crisis, are homeless, or are in inappropriate housing situations, including institutions.

A major intention of this project is to develop a permanent home for clients within a familiar and supportive community. The primary support for clients in this community is their peers. The primary task of staff is to support the functioning of the community as a whole. Specific treatment services, when needed, are provided by mental health program staff from other agencies. Project clients can live in this housing permanently without losing their homes if they need hospitalization or can be moved out if they become more stable. The goal of this project is to develop interdependent community living for people whose psychological distress or dysfunction persists despite treatment.

Vocational Programs

Supported Competitive Employment (SCE) Program for the Severely & Persistently Mentally Ill, Thresholds Research Institute, Chicago, Illinois. The goal of this project is to enable persons with severe and persistent mental illness to find and maintain community employment. This initiative came about in response to follow-up statistics obtained by the Thresholds Research Institute on its transitional employment program. It was found that most clients were not able to make the transition to totally independent employment, but most were able to make the transition into paid employment in competitive industry if ongoing supported services could be delivered in the work settings. It is these ongoing supportive services that the Supported Competitive Employment (SCE) project addresses.

The project synthesizes two service delivery models—the psychosocial model of psychiatric rehabilitation and the supported employment model of vocational rehabilitation—ensuring that clients receive needed ongoing support that will enable them to keep jobs in mainstream employment settings.

National Clubhouse Expansion Program, Fountain House, Inc., New York, New York. The National Clubhouse Expansion Program is designed to strengthen and expand the clubhouse model of psychiatric rehabilitation across the United States. This model of psychiatric rehabilitation engages the men and women who are members of the clubhouse in a wide range of restorative activities having to do with the operation of the clubhouse itself. Working side by side with staff and other members, members achieve a sense of belonging and being needed. Integral to well-developed clubhouse programs is the opportunity for members to go to work in commerce and industry through Transitional Employment, a system of part-time jobs in real work situations with real paychecks. Studies have shown that with ongoing support, the experience of Transitional Employment leads to regained confidence and aspiration, and many members go on to full-time employment. Clubhouse programs address issues of case management, housing, and social and educational needs and are a vital link for their members in securing needed psychiatric, pharmacological, and medical services. Membership is lifelong if desired, and all members are continually offered opportunities to achieve the highest possible level of functioning in the community.

During the 1970s, through a multi-year grant from the National Institute of Mental Health, Fountain House undertook a national training program to provide the opportunity for mental health professionals to learn this model of working with severely and chronically mentally ill men and women. This has resulted in the establishment of over 200 facilities seeking to implement the Fountain House model, in thirty-five states and the District of Columbia. This rapid proliferation and the increasing demand for training and technical assistance led to the establishment of the National Clubhouse Expansion Program, which aims to strengthen the existing network of clubhouses, establish new programs, expand the model to states where none exist, increase training opportunities, and expand the number of Transitional Employment slots.

Rural Projects

Acute Crisis Team (ACT), Pathways, Inc., Ashland, Kentucky. In Kentucky, as in several other states, low-income persons thought to need involuntary hospital treatment are frequently held in county jails during the initial part of the commitment process. This project provides immediate assessment and crisis intervention to the people who are placed in jail while awaiting court action regarding commitment. It offers these chronically mentally ill prisoners an opportunity for voluntary treatment rather than hospital commitment or staying in jail, when appropriate. When the voluntary treatment is accepted, it eliminates the need for that person to be involuntarily committed to the state hospital. Whether treatment is to be voluntary or involuntary, the project staff work for the patient's prompt removal from jail, reducing the psychologically damaging effects of being incarcerated.

Intervention by the Acute Crisis Team facilitates the use of community treatment options. The ACT staff removes clients from the jail as quickly as possible and connects them to the appropriate treatment option. In situations where hospitalization cannot be avoided, the project staff work to have the hospitalization take place in a community hospital rather than in the state hospital. In addition to giving immediate attention to persons jailed while awaiting the commitment process, the project staff consult with jail and law enforcement staff about other chronically mentally ill persons with whom they have contact. The goal in such involvements is to identify and locate these persons in an attempt at moving them toward mental health treatment as quickly as appropriate and possible. Project staff also involve themselves extensively with the families of the chronically mentally ill in developing a voluntary treatment plan that will be effective. This increases family awareness of community services and makes it more likely that families will turn to them in future crisis situations.

Piedmont Authority Residential & Supported Employment Services, Piedmont Area MH/MR & Substance Abuse Authority, Concord, North Carolina. The difficulty of providing low-cost, decent housing and marketable job skills for chronically mentally ill persons living independently is a national problem. This demonstration project aims to meet the housing and employment needs of seriously mentally ill citizens in the primarily rural areas of Cabarrus, Stanley, and Union Counties of North Carolina. The project trains long-term seriously mentally ill clients in housing remodeling skills—carpentry, painting, and so on—as they renovate and maintain houses that will then become their homes. The project is developing group homes and supervised rental housing for clients.

The project attempts to reduce to a minimum any problematic behavior through its close supervision of the client and to demonstrate to community citizens the capabilities of the mentally ill who are being adequately treated. As clients become trained and skilled in the renovation and maintenance of housing, the project strives to evolve into client-staffed, self-supporting businesses in areas such as building maintenance, furniture and appliance repair, and the like. Low-cost housing with minor remodeling needs is sought for rental to persons with serious mental illness. These clients are expected to involve themselves in the remodeling work on their own houses or on peer housing. They receive two months' free rent in exchange for each 120 hours of remodeling work performed. They are trained and supervised in their remodeling work by project staff.

The project addresses the communities' and families' concerns for the safety, support, and control of the seriously mentally ill individuals through intensive community case management. It provides incentive for landlords to rent to the serious long-term mentally ill by enhancing and maintaining their properties and using the properties as the medium for training clients. Finally, the project assists successful community employment and residential placements for clients by use of prideful aspects of self-help and increased autonomy.

Specialized Projects

Prepaid Medical Project, South Carolina Department of Mental Health, Columbia, South Carolina. The Department of Mental Health, in cooperation with the State Health and Human Services Finance Commission (the Medicaid agency) has developed a statewide demonstration involving chronically mentally ill Medicaid beneficiaries. The goal is to provide these individuals with a full range of mental health and physical health care in their home communities in order to avoid unnecessary admission to state Mental Health Department inpatient facilities.

This project is being carried out by eight of South Carolina's seventeen community mental health centers, all of which are administered by the Department of Mental Health. These centers receive payment (in advance) for the cost of mental health services to this population. Services include those provided by intensive case management teams. Services are being provided in the clients' natural environment with the team members providing case management, support, advocacy coaching, and medication monitoring. The case-management teams coordinate medical care with primary care physicians who are paid a monthly fee for serving as the providers and monitors of medical services to the chronically mentally ill. The team is also assisted by a consulting psychiatrist and uses all available community resources to assist the clients to achieve maximum independence while residing in the community.

Community Connections, Senior Health and Peer Counseling Center, Santa Monica, California. The overall aim of this project is to deliver a comprehensive spectrum of services responsive to the multiple needs of chronically mentally ill older adults. The project is based in a community mental health center serving seniors living in the west side of Los Angeles County. The services provided include psychological and psychiatric assessment and treatment, case management, and triage to the following services: (1) partial day care, (2) peer counseling, (3) structured volunteer experiences, and (4) health promotion/health education programs. Each client's treatment program is individually tailored. The project provides services to both mobile and homebound seniors and to persons who are homeless or at risk of being homeless.

The project involves extensive networking with other organizations and institutions (for example, the Department of Social Supportive Services, senior centers, local hospitals and medical clinics, community mental health facilities, food programs, board and care homes, and psychosocial service agencies). The project will attempt to demonstrate the ability to maintain chronically mentally ill seniors in the community, reduce the need for institutionalization, decrease isolation, improve functioning, and increase clients' own perceptions of being useful and worthwhile to themselves and others.

El Puente (The Bridge), Tropical Texas Center for MH and MR, Edinburg, Texas. This program serves a population that is predominantly Hispanic. Traditionally, Hispanics in the region have not used mental health services in trying to care for persons with chronic mental illness. This is so because of a number of factors including traditional beliefs about the causes and meaning of mental illness, a strong stigma associated with mental illness, and mistrust of mental health programs and professionals, who may lack knowledge about important areas of Hispanic culture.

El Puente is a family-support program designed to help the chronically mentally ill persons of the Lower Rio Grande Valley and their families deal with mental health problems through the use of a culturally sensitive and appropriate multifaceted treatment and training program. Program staff try to learn more about traditionally accepted cultural beliefs about mental illness and meld them with current scientific explanations. Their efforts focus on providing basic education regarding mental illness, its causes, methods of treatment, and appropriate coping strategies, to family members and clients. The goal is to develop an expanded frame of reference for explaining and dealing with problems associated with mental illness, so that Hispanics in this area will be more willing to participate in community-based treatment instead of relying solely on hospital treatment when things become unmanageable with the patient.

Educational/training programs are facilitated by staff who have been especially trained to be more culturally knowledgeable. They will attempt to demonstrate how various treatment approaches augment the family's traditional efforts in coping with mental illness. Educational programs for clients and families are provided in Spanish and English and in noninstitutional settings. Staff encourage the involvement of immediate family members, extended family, and significant others in an attempt to establish and provide a comprehensive supportive program of care for the seriously ill client. Major outreach efforts are being made to locate and bring into the program the chronically mentally ill who are not now being served in the community, and Community Service Aides provide augmented psychosocial programming during evenings and weekends.

Mental Health Nurse Preceptor Program, Providence Hospital, Anchorage, Alaska. The need for specialized care of the chronically mentally ill continues to grow in rural Alaska. Alarming increases have been noted in suicide rates and the numbers of chronically mentally ill among native Alaskans. These increases may be caused by a variety of factors, including the breakdown of traditional ways of life, the difficult commingling of two cultures, loneliness, or Alaskan natives' regret over the lack of control of their lives. Not surprisingly, native Americans admitted to the state hospital are overrepresented relative to the general population.

This project provides the opportunity for nurses in rural Alaska to become better trained in working with persons who have serious long-term mental illness. After being trained they return to their rural communities and provide assessment, intervention, treatment, and referral previously provided only in the state hospital. As a result, many of the persons now sent to the state hospital are able to remain in their own communities. Over an eighteen-month period, approximately thirty-six rural Alaskan nurses are spending a minimum of two weeks in training at Providence Hospital in Anchorage. They are working with mental health specialists, emergency room staff, and community service agencies to learn the mental health skills that will help them serve the residents needing services in their own communities.

Conclusion

Neglect of the chronically mentally ill living in our communities is a national disgrace and has been a media issue for several years. This neglect continues despite the knowledge to implement programs that significantly improve the quality of these individuals' lives. The reasons for our slowness in implementing these programs are multiple and include the resistance of mental health professionals to change the way they operate. It is clear from the projects described in this paper that mental health professionals need to relate to clients and to each other in ways that significantly differ from the traditional psychotherapeutic interventions. The paucity of programs, and thus the small numbers of professionals working within them, results in very little pressure for change coming from within the profession. One of the reasons the Mental Health Services Development Program is so important is that it is creating a significant number of innovative programs to serve the chronically mentally ill in a large number of communities. When the number of programs reaches a critical mass, movement will occur and set us on our way to ending the neglect of the chronically mentally ill.

References

Aiken, L. H., Somers, S. A., and Shore, M. F. "Private Foundations in Health Affairs." *American Psychologist,* 1986, *41* (11), 1290–1295.

Levit, K. R., Lazenby, H., Waldo, D. R., and Davidoff, L. M. "National Health Expenditures." *Health Care Financing Review,* 1985, *7,* 1–35.

Nielsen, W. A. *The Golden Donors: A New Anatomy of the Great Foundations.* New York: Dutton, 1985.

Robert Wood Johnson Foundation, annual report, 1987.

Leonard I. Stein is professor of psychiatry at the University of Wisconsin Medical School and director of the Mental Health Services Development Program, Madison, Wisconsin.

The authors discuss the benefits of including a research component in psychosocial programming and strategies for evaluating the outcomes and implementation of a rehabilitation program.

Integrating a Research Agenda into a New Psychosocial Rehabilitation Program

Freda Hansburg, Phyllis Solomon, Arthur T. Meyerson

Although many have cited the need for systematic evaluations of community support programs and their patient-client outcomes, research on the community treatment and rehabilitation of persons with serious mental illness remains limited. Obstacles to conducting such research have been well documented. Assessment of treatment outcomes has been complicated by a lack of consensually held operational definitions of rehabilitation and community support, disagreements over appropriate outcome measures, and methodological problems in applying experimental designs to clinical programs (Bachrach, 1982; Test and Stein, 1978; Schulberg, 1981; Brekke, 1988). The absence of research literature about program implementation makes it difficult to identify the ingredients of successful programs or to replicate program models (Brekke, 1988).

The "constituents" of psychosocial programs include members (patients-clients) and their families, administrators and staff, taxpayers, evaluators, funding sources and educators, all with legitimate claims to empirical data about what is or is not effective in helping persons with serious mental illness adjust to life in their communities. Determining program efficacy is essential for replication, program accountability, cost containment, and survival. Monitoring of program implementation is required to assess the extent to which our planned and operating programs are identical and to document barriers to program development. If we are to provide reliable answers to the question "What works for whom," the psychosocial rehabilitation field needs to develop research components with what appear to be effective programs (Meyerson and Herman, 1983).

One of the barriers to conducting research in psychosocial programs is the time-consuming nature of data collection. Most staff struggle to meet the demands of clinical work and paperwork and are thus resistant to research, which they experience as an added burden with little benefit or relevance to their work. They often feel that research is a separate endeavor, not within their clinical domain. The program director's perspective is likely to be that research is someone else's job, as program management is a full-time job. Our premise, however, is that research is intrinsic to effective management of a psychosocial program and enhancing to good clinical practice. We contend that program management is an exercise in action and operations research. Program directors continually make decisions, set goals, and plan initiatives in the hope that these actions will produce evidence of clinical and cost effectiveness. Similarly, service providers are confronted with decisions about a client's benefit from treatment and attainment of goals. Should the client, for example, move to the next, more demanding step in the treatment process? Any clinical program can be viewed as embodying the hypothesis that the program will produce beneficial effects for participants. By introducing a formal evaluation process, service providers and administrators move from this implicit hypothesis about what works to explicit questions, specific goals, and systematic methods to gather information for and about decision making. Research should, therefore, be systematic and intrinsic to program management.

The process of moving from an intuitive to an empirical mode of program evaluation has been described by Linhorst (1988), who introduced a research component into the social club of a psychosocial rehabilitation center. Staff of the program were directly involved in reexamining the purpose of the program and formulating specific goals to be measured. Patient members were involved in data collection. Linhorst noted that the evaluation process became "an integrated component" of the program, "providing a continual source of information" without producing time-management problems (p. 43). Linhorst's account suggests that different groups can benefit from program evaluation. Member involvement in the evaluation process provides an opportunity for consumer input into program development, conveys respect for consumers' perspectives, and reminds service providers that "keeping the customer satisfied" is important. Program evaluation can be a way to clarify program goals and reduce confusion about purposes and priorities for staff members. By becoming specific about program goals and their measurement, clinical staff can increase feedback about the outcomes of their clinical efforts. They may be rewarded by evaluation results that confirm successes and allow them to take note of small changes in clients that might otherwise go unidentified. Program directors can increase the amount of relevant information available before making management decisions. They are likely to feel more confident about continuing, introducing, or expanding program initiatives that are based on such information. They will find themselves better prepared to advocate for the continuance or expansion of the program with groups who have a legitimate need to assess cost effectiveness in order to determine funding, or to monitor service provision for purposes of licensure or accreditation status. Those desiring to replicate models or to assess the state of the art of psychosocial programming also need these data.

The inception of a new psychosocial rehabilitation program is a particularly opportune time to focus on a research agenda. Incorporation of an evaluation process into the initial program implementation creates a base for addressing future research questions. The integration of program design and program evaluation facilitates planning, as both activities require specificity of program purpose, goals, and methodology. The staff of the new program gain a better understanding of the intended model when program elements are stated in the observable and measurable terms essential for monitoring implementation.

Starting a new program involves setting norms that will powerfully influence individual and group performance. Integrating the evaluation process into the program from the beginning helps orient staff to the importance of research and desensitizes them to dealing with forms and to having aspects of their performance monitored. This can convey a message that their work will be taken seriously. Establishing the program as a vehicle for future research can create an *esprit de corps* by the recognition that the team will be contributors to rather than passive participants in the development of their own program, and possibly contributors to the field.

An Example: IMPACT

IMPACT (Independent Mastery: Psychosocial Approaches to Community Treatment) is a psychiatric rehabilitation/day treatment program that operates as a component of Hahnemann University's new Ambulatory Psychiatric Services. Licensed as a partial hospital by the Office of Mental Health of the Commonwealth of Pennsylvania, IMPACT began providing integrated clinical and rehabilitation programming for adults with moderate to severe mental illness in February of 1989. The mission of IMPACT is to enable its members to be successful and satisfied in community living, learning, and working environments of their choice. One of the major goals of the program is to reduce rates of psychiatric hospitalization among members.

The IMPACT program combines clinical modalities such as psychiatric evaluation and pharmacological therapy, psychological therapy, psychological testing, and group psychotherapy with psychosocial rehabilitation approaches, including functional assessment, direct skills teaching, case management, and prevocational training. Members are taught needed skills in such areas as communication and problem solving, symptom and stress management, job-seeking, and activities of daily living. Psychoeducational workshops dealing with the management of mental illness are offered to members' families, and a "Double Trouble" group provides peer counseling and support to members who have substance abuse problems associated with their psychiatric disorders.

The philosophy of IMPACT is that rehabilitation is done *with* people, not to them, and to that end member choice and involvement are emphasized throughout the treatment process. Staff, who are mental health professionals at master's and bachelor's degree levels, are provided with in-service training in rehabilitation technology and communication skills designed to maximize client participation in setting goals, identifying functional strengths and deficits, and developing individual rehabilitation plans.

Program Model. The program model used at IMPACT is based on the psychiatric rehabilitation approach developed by Anthony and Associates at the Center for Psychiatric Rehabilitation at Boston University. Psychiatric rehabilitation is essentially a psychoeducational process; a specific and replicable technology to assist persons with a psychiatric disability in mastering the skills required to live, learn, or work in their communities with a minimum of support from the mental health system (Anthony, 1979). Based on the model of impairment, disability, and handicap underlying the field of physical rehabilitation, psychiatric rehabilitation practice focuses on maximizing the adaptive functioning of the individual within his or her chosen setting. This is accomplished by enhancing needed skill performance or modifying the environment to make it more supportive of the individual's level of function (Rogers, Anthony, and Jansen, 1988). A rehabilitation diagnosis in this model includes an overall rehabilitation goal (a decision about where the patient intends to live, learn, or work) and a functional and resource assessment (that is, an evaluation of the skills and supports the individual has and needs in order to meet his or her overall rehabilitation goal). Rehabilitation plans specify who will do what to overcome the identified skill and resource deficits. Rehabilitation interventions focus on skill and resource development. Direct skills teaching is provided when patients need to acquire specific competencies, whereas skill-use programs provide step-by-step action plans to assist patients in applying their skills in appropriate settings. Resource coordination includes interventions designed to link patients with needed people, places, things, and activities (Anthony, Cohen, and Farkas, 1982). The availability of standardized modules for training personnel in the skills of psychiatric rehabilitation facilitates replication of these techniques across programs.

There is an emerging data base to support the efficacy of the psychiatric rehabilitation approach. Dion and Anthony (1987) have reviewed the outcomes of over thirty experimental and quasi-experimental research studies addressing psychiatric rehabilitation interventions. They conclude that these interventions are associated with positive outcomes, including decreased recidivism, increased community tenure, increased rates of client employment and productivity, increased skill development and satisfaction, and decreased costs.

Client Characteristics. Located in center-city Philadelphia, IMPACT is accessible by public transportation and serves a population that is primarily urban and low income. Referrals to the program have come primarily from Hahnemann's three adult psychiatric inpatient units (53 percent), with the balance referred by Hahnemann outpatient clinics and other community sources, including family members, mental health programs, and private practitioners. As of May 1989, a total of forty-one individuals have been accepted as referrals to IMPACT, thirty-six of whom have been seen for initial (intake) evaluation. An analysis of those evaluated for the program indicated that 60 percent were women and 40 percent men. Twenty-nine percent of IMPACT candidates were caucasian, 60 percent were black, and the rest were about half Hispanic and half Asian. Candidates ranged in age from 19 to 57, with the mean age being 31.6. The vast majority of candidates (92 percent) are adults in their twenties and thirties.

In terms of severity of illness, IMPACT candidates are consistent with the National Institute of Mental Health criteria for moderate to severe mental illness. Fifty-three percent have a primary psychiatric diagnosis of schizophrenia or schizoaffective disorder, 32 percent a diagnosis of affective or mood disorder, 12 percent a primary diagnosis of personality disorder, and the remaining 3 percent have deferred or other diagnoses. Among the individuals evaluated at IMPACT, 86 percent have a history of psychiatric hospitalization and 46 percent have a current problem or history of substance abuse.

Overview of Research Agenda and Process. The proposed research agenda for IMPACT needed to encompass two essential components: a program-monitoring evaluation and a client-outcome evaluation. The process evaluation, or monitoring, was considered necessary for documenting the actual clinical and rehabilitation services that are delivered to members as well as for determining whether the program is implemented as originally intended. Research data will be the basis for providing appropriate feedback to the administrator and staff on what corrective actions need to be taken. The evaluation of outcome will enable the determination of the program's degree of efficacy. These data will provide information to assist in program justification and, we hope, will contribute new knowledge to the field of psychiatric rehabilitation.

Overview

Preparing Staff for Research Activities. In establishing a new psychosocial program, we were afforded the luxury of incorporating research expectations into the initial personnel recruitment and hiring process. A research value orientation was a major consideration in the hiring of the new director. The program manager sets a model for other program staff involved in implementing the research (Brekke, 1988). As part of a new emphasis in the Department of Mental Health Sciences, a full-time experienced researcher was hired who has a commitment to evaluating the psychiatric rehabilitation of severely mentally disabled persons. This provided a research consultant to the program.

The newly hired director of the psychosocial program was aware that without the commitment of the program staff, the research agenda would probably not be implemented successfully. Research expectations were specified in the recruitment interviews in order to ensure the full cooperation of program staff in the research efforts. Job descriptions included research functions, such as data collection. An assessment of the applicant's willingness to participate in these efforts was a component of the hiring decision. Staff orientation and training included instruction in the use of standardized behavioral symptom and social function rating scales that were selected as a component of the ongoing assessment of members. Since two of the staff were certified by Boston University as qualified trainers in psychiatric rehabilitation technology, in-service training in the planned program model could be readily implemented with new staff. A Rehabilitation Facts and Values Survey (developed by the Center for Psychiatric Rehabilitation, Boston University) was administered to staff on the first day of their employment in order to measure their initial knowledge of and attitudes toward psychiatric rehabilitation and the target population. Pre- and post-tests of staff skill levels were incorporated into the initial training. The use of standardized training packages produced by the Center for Psychiatric Rehabilitation facilitated quality control in the training curriculum.

Initial Evaluation Questions. The initial step in the research process was the development of some basic research questions concerning the psychiatric rehabilitation program. These were developed by the program manager and reviewed by the research consultant. The research consultant made minor revisions to ensure that the questions were stated in researchable terms. These questions can be categorized in three general areas: (1) Patient Descriptions and Outcomes, (2) Patients' Actual Use of and Experience with the Program, and (3) Program Description and Monitoring.

Examples of the types of research questions generated follow.

Patient/Consumer Descriptions and Outcomes.

1. What are the demographic and clinical characteristics of IMPACT members?
2. To what extent do IMPACT members show functional changes at six months, one year, and two years after admission? Specifically,
   a. Is there an increase in the proportion of members working or looking for work after six months, one year, and two years? Among those working, is there an increase in earned income and average number of hours worked per week?
   b. To what extent have members moved to more independent living arrangements?
   c. To what extent is there a decrease in the average number of inpatient days and emergency room contacts among members at six months, one year, and two years after admission? How do these statistics compare to six months and one year prior to admission?
   d. To what extent do members show increased level-of-functioning scores? Decrease in psychiatric symptoms?
   e. Is there a decrease in the number or severity ratings (or both) of symptoms reported or observed among members?
   f. Do members show increased medication adherence at six months, one year, and two years?
3. Do demographic, clinical, or environmental factors discriminate members who improve in work status, living arrangements, use of inpatient days, emergency room contacts, social functioning, reduction of symptoms, and medication adherence from those who do not improve?
4. What is the degree of agreement on ratings of members' level of social functioning at intake and discharge among the members, IMPACT staff, and members' families or significant others? Is there a greater degree of agreement at discharge than at intake?

Patients-Consumers Use of Program.

1. What is the frequency of members' attendance at IMPACT?
2. What is the length of stay at IMPACT?
3. What proportion of candidates referred to IMPACT are admitted?
4. What proportion of IMPACT admissions graduate from the program (that is, move on to successful functioning in their chosen community settings)?
5. Are there demographic, clinical, or environmental factors that discriminate among the following subgroups?
   a. IMPACT graduates
   b. IMPACT dropouts
   c. IMPACT members terminated before graduation
   d. Candidates not admitted to IMPACT.

Program Description and Monitoring.

1. What is the average number of treatment days required to develop each of the following:
   a. Overall Rehabilitation Goal
   b. Functional Assessment
   c. Comprehensive Resource Assessment
   d. Comprehensive Treatment Plan
   e. Skill-Use Program
   f. Community Resource Referral.
2. What proportion of the IMPACT members served have each of the following Overall Rehabilitation Goals?
   a. Stay at current living environment
   b. Stay at current work environment
   c. Stay at current educational environment
   d. Move to new living environment
   e. Move to new work environment
   f. Move to new educational environment.
3. What are the most frequent community survival skills and deficits identified by members' functional assessments?
4. How does the overall level of functioning relate to strengths and deficits in skills identified by the functional assessment?
5. What are the most frequent support strengths and deficits identified by members' comprehensive resource assessments?
6. What are the average number of skill and resource-development goals listed in members' Comprehensive Treatment Plans? What is the frequency distribution of the ratios of skill-development to resource-development goals?
7. What proportion of Comprehensive Treatment Plans include Direct Skill Teaching as an intervention?
8. To what extent do skill-use ratings correspond to needed skill performance levels identified in the functional assessment?
9. To what extent does the number of treatment days required to implement a skill-use program differ when the member came with knowledge of a skill or learned the skill at IMPACT?
10. To what extent do community resource referrals correspond to Overall Rehabilitation Goals?
11. To what extent do IMPACT Entry, Success, (that is, meeting specified criteria for maximum benefit from the program) and Exit Skill ratings predict graduation from IMPACT and achievement of Overall Rehabilitation Goals?
12. Is there an increase in the number of *skill lesson plans* (that is, detailed plans for direct skill teaching) in program files six months, one year, and two years after program inception?
13. Is there an increase in the number of affiliation agreements devel-

oped with other providers six months, one year, and two years after program inception?

14. Is there an increase in the types and quality of placements to which members are referred one year and two years after program inception?

15. Is there an increase in ratings of staff skills in conducting rehabilitation diagnosis, planning, and intervention six months, one year, and two years after program inception?

A clearly delineated set of data emerges as a result of formulating this initial set of research questions. These data elements then provide direction for the nature of the intake and discharge forms as well as for the program monitoring forms that are an essential component of the data base.

Developing a Monitoring Plan and Data Base. Creating a plan for monitoring the implementation and outcomes of IMPACT services is an ongoing objective of the new program. Although psychiatric rehabilitation technology lends itself to monitoring because of its specificity, the development of monitoring systems can be a formidable task in any program. Forms used for program monitoring must be convenient and adaptive to ensure their continued use while satisfying requirements of reliability and validity. The availability of such tools remains limited in clinical practice. At IMPACT, although we have selected some of the tools we will use to monitor program implementation and outcome, we recognize that other instruments need to be identified or developed to facilitate the evaluation process.

In order to monitor program outcome, it is necessary to record and describe the progress of consumers as they enter, use, and leave the IMPACT program. Demographic and clinical information is gathered at intake. This includes treatment, residential, educational, and vocational history. Throughout clients' participation, their levels of functioning and symptomatology are assessed at specified intervals. Functioning is presently rated by staff using the Specific Level of Functioning scale (Schneider and Struening, 1983); and client's symptoms are rated by the patient's psychiatric resident-physicians, using the Brief Psychiatric Rating Scale (Overall and Gorham, 1962). These scales were selected because they had relatively high reliability and validity and could be easily completed by program staff. These instruments are of reasonable length and merely require checking the appropriate responses. Selection of scales for program monitoring requires consideration of staff time and skill as well as research requirements. Some scales are reliable and valid for research purposes but are too time consuming and demanding to be completed by program staff on an ongoing basis. Data sheets have been developed to summarize and aggregate information about consumers during and after their participation in the program. Such information includes diagnosis, symptom, and skill ratings and types of resources needed. These monitoring forms are presently being used in a pilot project: an initial, six-month analysis of the IMPACT population.

Evaluation of program implementation at IMPACT is facilitated by using the ubiquitous "pink worksheets" that are completed with consumers during Primary Rehabilitation groups in the program. The worksheets include forms for developing overall rehabilitation goals, conducting functional assessments, programming skill use, and other components of psychiatric rehabilitation technology. Also included are IMPACT Entry, Success, and Exit Skill assessments that are completed with consumers as they move through Candidate, Member, and Graduate phases of the program, respectively. A Resource Assessment is also completed at each phase of the cycle. Since the worksheets are intrinsic to the program, they are implemented routinely in designated groups and provide an ongoing source of data for program decisions.

A recent review showed that approximately two-thirds of the IMPACT population are working toward moving to new vocational and educational settings, and the remaining third are concentrating on moving to new living environments or succeeding at their current residential setting. This information prompted the program to introduce more hours of prevocationally oriented programming to clients during Primary Rehabilitation group. Similarly, Linhorst (1988) used information from a client survey to introduce more special-interest groups in his psychosocial program. The results of a consumer-satisfaction survey being implemented at IMPACT will be tracked using the previously mentioned data sheets and analyzed as part of the initial six-month evaluation process. A data base of the major variables for both process and outcome evaluation scales is being created. These data will be entered into the computer on a continuous basis. Elements include client demographics, clinical characteristics, and outcomes.

Specialized Research Projects. Another aspect of the research agenda is the development of more specialized research efforts that emerge as the psychosocial program is implemented. These research activities tend to be more complex and require additional resources. Research projects will be submitted to governmental funding agencies, that is, NIMH and private foundations. An example is a proposal submitted to the National Institute on Disability and Rehabilitation Research Innovations Grants Program. The grant was titled "Compliance with Referrals to a Psychosocial Rehabilitation Program: Mental Health Consumer vs. Professional Linkage Strategies."

The idea for this research project was generated by a need to increase attendance at the program. This proposed research will assess the efficacy of employing mental health consumers as linking agents to the program by conducting outreach, intake, and continuance procedures for other clients versus having professionals conduct these same procedures. Another aspect of this proposal is to determine whether these mental health consumers who function as linking agents have increased self-esteem and social functioning and decreased behavioral symptomatology. A third aspect of the project will be to assess whether the psychiatric inpatient unit staff have more positive views of the rehabilitation capabilities of psychiatric patients after having the opportunity of observing consumers in such a linkage role.

Some of these outreach efforts were being done by professionals before submission of the grant. The proposed research will afford us an opportunity to experiment with different outreach strategies and also to systematize and refine efforts that were already being employed.

In the future, we foresee developing research proposals in several areas, including the extent to which skills learned in a psychosocial rehabilitation program generalize to other settings, and which staff characteristics result in more effective rehabilitation outcomes. As the program develops, new experimental service components will emerge that can be added to the program and evaluated with new research efforts. Thus a research agenda may stimulate new and innovative services.

Conclusion

In an environment of scarce resources, there is an increasing emphasis on program accountability. As IMPACT's experience suggests, a research agenda can be introduced into a psychosocial program that becomes, as a result, systematic and explicit about its goals and objectives. Incorporating a research component creates a basis for rational program-development decisions, quality assurance, and program advocacy efforts and helps contribute new knowledge to the field of psychiatric rehabilitation.

A program administrator can introduce an evaluation component by identifying existing instruments to measure progress toward the goals and objectives set forth for patients in the program. Where such tools are unavailable, program directors and staff, with research consultation, can develop evaluation instruments. Although these may not meet the research criteria of reliability and validity, they will provide systematic data on which to base better program decisions. Over time, the validity and reliability of such instruments can then be assessed. Complicated or specialized studies may require more intense involvement or technical assistance from the experienced research personnel. Vehicles such as NIMH's P.A.L. (Public Academic Liaison) initiative can serve as incentives for academic researchers who require clinical populations to work with clinical programs in designing research studies and grant proposals. Graduate students at the dissertation level may also be involved in research consultation and efforts. In some states, technical assistance for research may be available through the State Office of Mental Health. Time, effort, and financial resources invested in research endeavors should provide the data that will make decisions more efficacious and less time consuming. Research takes time, but it should save time and resources in the long run.

References

Anthony, W. *Principles of Psychiatric Rehabilitation.* Baltimore: University Park Press, 1979.

Anthony, W., Cohen, M., and Farkas, M. "A Psychiatric Rehabilitation Treatment Program: Can I Recognize One If I See One?" *Community Mental Health Journal,* 1982, *18,* 83–95.

Bachrach, L. "Assessment of Outcomes in Community Support Systems: Results, Problems, and Limitations." *Schizophrenia Bulletin,* 1982, *8* (1), 39–60.

Brekke, J. "What Do We Really Know About Community Support Programs? Strategies for Better Monitoring." *Hospital and Community Psychiatry,* 1988, *39* (9), 946–952.

Dion, G., and Anthony, W. "Research in Psychiatric Rehabilitation: A Review of Experimental and Quasi-Experimental Studies." *Rehabilitation Counseling Bulletin,* 1987, *30,* 177–203.

Linhorst, D. "The Development of a Program Evaluation System for Psychosocial Rehabilitation Centers." *Psychosocial Rehabilitation Journal,* 1988, *12* (2), 35–43.

Meyerson, A., and Herman, G. "What's New in Aftercare: A Review of Recent Literature." *Hospital and Community Psychiatry,* 1983, *34,* 333–342.

Overall, J., and Gorham, D. "The Brief Psychiatric Rating Scale." *Psychological Reports,* 1962, *10,* 799–812.

Rogers, E., Anthony, W., and Jansen, M. "Psychiatric Rehabilitation as One Preferred Response to the Needs of Individuals with Severe Psychiatric Disability." *Rehabilitation Psychology,* 1988, *33* (1), 5–14.

Schneider, L., and Struening, E. "SLOF: A Rating Scale for Assessing the Mentally Ill." *Social Work Research and Abstracts,* 1983, *19,* 9–21.

Schulberg, H. "Outcome Evaluations in the Mental Health Field." *Community Mental Health Journal,* 1981, *17* (2), 132–142.

Test, M., and Stein, L. "Community Treatment of the Chronic Patient: Research Overview." *Schizophrenia Bulletin,* 1978, *4* (3), 350–364.

Freda Hansburg is director of IMPACT and senior instructor in the Department of Mental Health Sciences, Hahnemann University.

Phyllis Solomon is director of the Section of Mental Health Services and Systems Research and professor, Department of Mental Health Sciences, Hahnemann University.

Arthur T. Meyerson is chair and professor of the Department of Mental Health Sciences, Hahnemann University.

INDEX

Ordering Information

New Directions for Mental Health Services is a series of paperback books that presents timely and readable volumes on subjects of concern to clinicians, administrators, and others involved in the care of the mentally disabled. Each volume is devoted to one topic and includes a broad range of authoritative articles written by noted specialists in the field. Books in the series are published quarterly in Fall, Winter, Spring and Summer, and are available for purchase by subscription as well as by single copy.

Subscriptions for 1990 cost $48.00 for individuals (a savings of 20 percent over single-copy prices) and $64.00 for institutions, agencies, and libraries. Please do not send institutional checks for personal subscriptions. Standing orders are accepted.

Single copies cost $14.95 when payment accompanies order. (California, New Jersey, New York, and Washington, D.C., residents please include appropriate sales tax.) Billed orders will be charged postage and handling.

Discounts for quantity orders are available. Please write to the address below for information.

All orders must include either the name of an individual or an official purchase order number. Please submit your order as follows:

Subscriptions: specify series and year subscription is to begin

Single copies: include individual title code (such as MHS1)

Mail all orders to:

Jossey-Bass Inc., Publishers
350 Sansome Street
San Francisco, California 94104

Other Titles Available in the New Directions for Mental Health Services Series

H. Richard Lamb, Editor-in-Chief